KV-190-766

PERSPECTIVES VOLUME 2:
PHYSICAL ACTIVITY AND AGEING

Contributing Authors

Steve Bailey (Editor)

Dr. Bailey holds a Bachelor of Education degree in Physical Education and English and a PhD in History (Physical Education). He has been a teacher of physical education for 19 years and was Director of Physical Education at Winchester College, England, for ten years. He has published and presented papers at conferences on: the modern Olympic Games, secondary physical education, sports history, technology in physical education. Books published include: 'Science in the Service of Physical Education and Sport'; 'Readings in Sports History'; and '100 Years of Physical Education 1899-1999'. He is currently contracted to write the History of the Paralympic Movement.

Patricia Vertinsky

Dr. Patricia Vertinsky is Professor and Head of the Department of Educational Studies at the University of British Columbia. She is the President of the North American Sport History Association (NASSH), Board member of ISHPES, and an International Fellow of the American Academy of Kinesiology and Physical Education. She is a social and cultural historian of health, physical activity and sport with a particular focus upon representations of the body. Her many publications include The *Eternally Wounded Woman: Doctors, Women and Exercise in the Late Nineteenth Century*, and her research has focused upon a multi-faceted study of the

Correspondence regarding *Perspectives*: ICSSPE/CIEPSS, Am Kleinen Wannsee 6, 14109 Berlin, Germany. Tel: +49 30 805 00360 Fax: +49 30 805 6386 E-mail:icsspe@icsspe.org ageing female body in exercise and sports, the marking of race and gender upon the body, and most recently, disability, normalcy and the body.

Don Bailey

Professor Don Bailey has been a faculty member in the College of Kinesiology at the University of Saskatchewan in Canada since 1959, assuming the position of Professor Emeritus in 1994. Since 1994, he has been a Visiting Professor at the University of Queensland in Australia for six months each year. Among his research accomplishments, Professor Bailey was the Director of the Saskatchewan Child Growth and Development Study during the 1960's and 70's. Results of this 10-year longitudinal investigation of growth and fitness in children have had an important impact on school programs of health and physical education in Canada and abroad. For the past number of years he has been involved in studying the effects of weight-bearing physical activity on bone mineral acquisition and skeletal integrity in children. Currently, he is the principal investigator of the widely recognised longitudinal Saskatchewan Pediatric Bone Mineral Accrual Study started in 1991. The results of his research have been published in numerous medical and scientific journals around the world. Currently he is Vice President of the International Council for Physical Activity and Fitness Research (ICPAFR).

Michael Sagiv

Professor Michael Sagiv is the Head of the Wingate College in Israel. He obtained his Doctorate at the University of Wisconsin, USA, and was also a professor at the Medical School, Department of Physiology and Pharmacology of Tel Aviv University. Currently, Dr. Sagiv is the President of the European Group for Research into Elderly and Physical Activity, a Fellow of the American College of Sports Medicine, a member of the Israeli Academy of Physical Education, Head of the Sports Medicine Committee of Israel Athletic Association and a member of the World Health Organisation's Committee on Ageing. Dr. Sagiv contributes to the scientific field as an invited speaker regularly at international and national meetings and is an editorial board member of four refereed journals. He has published 66 referred articles and numerous book chapters and other publications.

Perspectives - The Multidisciplinary Series of
Physical Education and Sport Science
Volume 2, October 2000

PHYSICAL ACTIVITY AND AGEING

Contents

Sandra Matsudo

Sandra Mahecha Matsudo is General Director of the Physical Fitness Research Center in São Caetano do Sul (CELAFISCS), São Paulo, Brazil, and Scientific Advisor of the Agita São Program funded by the State Secretary of Health of São Paulo. CELAFISCS was awarded an International Award of Sports Medicine in the Olympic Games in Barcelona 1992, and the Prince Faizal International Award of the International Federation of Physical Education (FIEP) in 1996. She is a physician and is finishing her PhD in Sports Medicine at the Federal University of São Paulo. Her research interests lie in the fields of ageing and physical activity and physical activity promotion. She has authored and co-authored almost 50 publications in paediatric exercise, ageing and physical fitness and the promotion of physical activity. She is the executive editor of the *Brazilian Journal of Science and Movement* and an editorial board member of five Brazilian journals of physical education. Dr. Matsudo is the Chair of the Longitudinal Physical Fitness and Aging Project in São Caetano do Sul.

Michael Kolb

Michael Kolb studied Physical Education and German at Karlsruhe University, Germany. After two years of teaching at a high school he began work as a scientific collaborator at the German University of Sports and Sport Sciences in Cologne, where he was a member of the Department of Pedagogy from 1983 - 1991. In 1989, he completed his PhD on "Play as a phenomenon - the phenomenon of play" in Sport Pedagogy and Sport Philosophy. In 1992, he moved to the Department for Sport and Sport Sciences at Kiel University where he worked as a scientific collaborator and was qualified to lecture in Sport Sciences in 1998. His Habilitation (a required post-doctorate thesis) focused on: "Motivated Ageing. Perspectives of Sport Educational Gerontology" and it received an award in the Carl-Diem-Contest, the most important contest for sport sciences in Germany.

His main fields of research are sport educational gerontology; pedagogic and didactic aspects of play, sport and games; methods of body perception and relaxation; and possibilities for health promotion, prevention and rehabilitation via physical activity.

Maaret Ilmarinen

Maaret Ilmarinen graduated in Physical Education at the University of Jyväskylä and in Sports Information Science at the University of Helsinki, Finland. She is the Project Manager at the Research Center for Sport and Health Sciences, LIKES, implementing a national "Fit for Life" programme (1995 – 2004). Additionally, she has worked for the Finnish Society for Research in Sport and Physical Education and the Ministry of Education (1979 – 1994) implementing national and international projects, seminars and congresses. She has edited several related publications including: *Stronger through Physical Exercise, Social Justification of Sport, Sport and International Understanding, Planning the Future of Sport* (from the corresponding Congress of the Council of Europe). As a secretary for the parliamentary Sports Committee she produced the national sports strategy for 1990-1999. She has been a member of the group of sports information scientists of the Council of Europe and the ICSSPE Editorial Board. From 1975 – 1979, at the Information Service for Sport and Health Sciences at LIKES Research Center in Jyväskylä she edited scientific abstracts from all areas of sport research and trained sports students in information science.

C. Jessie Jones

Jessie Jones, Professor in the Division of Kinesiology and Health Promotion, Director of the Lifespan Wellness Clinic, Co-director of the Center for Successful Aging, and Coordinator of Gerontology Programs at California State University, Fullerton (CSUF), has an extensive background in gerontology and exercise science and ageing. Most recently, Dr. Jones has been appointed as the Director of Programs and Research for the Overseas Chinese Institute on Aging.

Professor Jones is nationally and internationally known in the field of exercise science and ageing for her research, programme design, curriculum development, and instructor training. In addition to being the recipient of several research grants and honour awards for her work related to the prevention of diseases and disability and the promotion of successful ageing, Dr. Jones' work has been published in numerous professional journals, cited in over a hundred popular newspapers and magazines, and presented at various conferences across the U.S. and abroad.

Roberta E. Rikli

Roberta Rikli is a professor and chair of the Division of Kinesiology and Health Promotion at California State University, Fullerton and is Co-Director of the LifeSpan National Assessment Project. Dr. Rikli has long-term teaching and research interests in the field of measurement and evaluation and in older adult fitness. Her work in this field has led to numerous invitations to speak at conferences and workshops throughout the nation and abroad. She has published numerous articles and abstracts which have appeared in journals such as the *Research Quarterly for Exercise and Sport, Journal of Gerontology, Journal of Experimental and Clinical Gerontology, Journal of Aging and Physical Activity, Journal of Physical Education, Recreation and Dance, Medicine and Science in Sports and Exercise, and Measurement in Physical Education and Exercise Science*, and her work has also been cited in hundreds of popular press magazines and journals.

PERSPECTIVES VOLUME 2:
PHYSICAL ACTIVITY AND AGEING

Editorial

Steve Bailey

"Old folks have ambitions and dreams, too, like everybody else and why don't they work for them? Why don't they go for it? Don't sit on a couch someplace, that's my attitude."
(Senator John Glenn, on his recent return from a mission into space)

Ageing has many different meanings in different contexts: a growing child acquires new skills and an understanding of its world; we mature into adulthood and begin to take responsibility for our actions and their impact on others; and we reach a point in our development when we are perceived to have a declining capacity for valuable contribution to the society we have helped to build and maintain. It is this third 'age' that this collection of papers relates to. This is a collection of papers about the need to empower the population of older adults, to replace myth with facts based on systematic research about physical capacity and positive prevention. It is a chance to identify the problem of taking for granted the assumptions of past generations that the elderly do not require as much attention to their sporting opportunities because they are in 'years of decline'! Above all, it is a selection of papers that sets out a vocabulary for sports scientists to renew discussions about physical activity and ageing that may take place between disciplines – for it is the stated aim of this book series to open up pathways so that historically entrenched academic disciplines can feel at ease crossing subject boundaries and sharing possibilities that may just make a difference to the target population.

Correspondence to: Dr. Steve Bailey, Director of Physical Education, Winchester College, Morshead's, 33 Cross Road, SO23 9JA Winchester, United Kingdom

"Age wrinkles the body. Quitting wrinkles the soul"
(Douglas MacArthur)

In early cultures decisions of any importance were put before assemblies of elders, wise persons (then predominantly men) who drew on past experience to see the continuity of the traditions of their community and who were entrusted with the maintenance of stability and harmony. The value to society was undoubted, even though these elders might no longer be regularly advancing the income or productivity of the group – they were respected as having moved into matriarchal/patriarchal roles, just as important as any previous contribution they may have made. The community owed these older adults a debt of service and reverence, and they were looked after with tenderness.

As we have moved away from a societal model of nuclear families with home-based enterprise we have also altered the value attached to older members of society. Many more people live some distance away from their immediate families, and the elderly who live alone must make a greater effort in order to enjoy these years. It is common for people to pursue earlier retirement from full time employment, giving a greater number of years than before for them to participate in the numerous recreational opportunities that municipal authorities are carefully and considerately providing. But there is much to do before this simple equation (more years of retirement = more opportunity + more enjoyment by elderly) can be fulfilled. We need to persuade older adults not to comply with society's expectation that the elderly should just fade away – gradually losing faculties, becoming of less use but more of a drain to society.

"You can't reach old age by another man's road. My habits protect my life but they would assassinate you"
(Mark Twain, on his 70th birthday in 1905)

The route towards a suitable positive approach to ageing and physical activity should be concerned with giving legitimacy and opportunity back to the elderly, to encourage involvement and inclusion, to educate and to coax. They should be empowered to make a difference for themselves. There is a basic positive cost saving for community health programmes that can be used as an incentive to encourage municipal authorities to develop better facilities and opportunities.

Pat Vertinsky's paper is a worthy opening for this collection; she traces changing attitudes and meanings of ageing as the demographic shift has brought us a greater number of active adults enjoying 'the sunshine of their life'. Providing a historical foundation for understanding this collection of papers, Vertinsky visits areas not explored enough in sports history. The automatic association of sport with youth and vigour has tended against the building of elderly role models, and this has affected the promotional aspect of physical activity for an increasingly elderly population.

In a departure from the obvious focus of physical activity and ageing Don Bailey writes about physical activity and osteoporosis. The accepted fact that heredity features strongly is put alongside research that indicates the importance of physical activity as a preventative measure against the onset of osteoporosis. Bailey's paper gives equal importance to the place of physical activity in early life as for the elderly; prevention in a wider population, and compensatory action for hereditary determinism will help towards a healthier community, more physically active and able to enjoy life to the full.

Michael Sagiv examines the physiological effects on the body as it gets older. Maximum oxygen uptake and cardiac function are discussed in terms of changing training effects with ageing. It is encouraging to find out that there is a physiological basis for supporting extended physical training for older adults.

The particular problems encountered in developing countries are investigated by Sandra Matsudo, with a particular eye on Brazil. Far from stating the obvious, her paper demonstrates that there are many barriers to participation in physical activity by older adults in developing countries – not all dependent on low income or scarce facilities. This case study helps stress the wider relevance of holistic approaches to problems such as encouraging physical activity in elderly populations.

Michael Kolb's discussion looks at the areas of motivation and objective-setting. He makes suggestions for positive policy-making by those responsible for establishing programmes for physical activity among the elderly.

Programmes for physical activity in the elderly population of Finland have been examined by Maaret Ilmarinen. Various policies and programmes are discussed, and Ilmarinen gives a full picture of possibilities and directions for the future.

Roberta Rikli and Jesse Jones have reported in their paper on the need for functional assessment as an essential part of helping the worthwhile guidance of elderly in communities. Work at the Lifespan Wellness Clinic at California State University, Fullerton, has given them a setting for the establishment of a functional fitness test for older adults.

The writers in this book explain that much can be done – much is already being done – but that we have a long way to go before we will be giving the elderly their real due care and respect. This must involve carefully monitored physical activity for the maintenance of physical strength and well-being, for the prevention of onset of disorders known to affect older inactive adults, and to help stimulate mentally and socially so as to give satisfaction and pleasure to elderly people living life to the full.

"Age does not protect you from love.
But love, to some extent, protects you from age"
(Jeanne Moreau)

PERSPECTIVES VOLUME 2:
PHYSICAL ACTIVITY AND AGEING

Commentary

Irene Hoskins, Katja Borodulin,
World Health Organization

The global population of our planet is becoming older. In only 25 years the total population of older people (aged 60 and over) will increase from 605 million in the year 2000 to 1.2 billion in 2025. In a number of developed countries, there are already today more people aged 60 and over than there are children under 15. But while population ageing is already fairly well understood and much discussed in the developed world, it is not as readily recognised that it is in the developing world that we will see the steepest increases in the overall numbers of the aged, as well as the highest increases in the proportions of older persons making up societies. Already 60 % of older people live in the developing world now. By 2025 it will be more than 70 %. In some of the mega-countries in the developing world, such as China, Brazil and Nigeria, the populations of older people will double or even more than double in the next 25 years. Percentages of the older population in the total population of such countries will also increase considerably. For example, it took 114 years in France for the older population to increase from 7 % to 14 %. The same doubling will occur in China in less than 30 years.

As people live longer everywhere, it is of paramount importance for individuals to maintain independence and quality of life as they age. Research on the prevention of functional decline, premature morbidity and mortality now shows substantial evidence of the benefits of physical

Correspondence to: Ms. Irene Hoskins, Department for Health Promotion, Non-Communicable Disease Prevention, and Surveillance, World Health Organization, 20 Avenue Appia, 1211 Geneva 27, Switzerland activities throughout the life span as well as at older ages. Research tells us that being active reduces the risk of such non-communicable diseases as: heart disease, obesity, hypertension, diabetes, osteoporosis, depression as well as falls and injuries.

Among older persons, health gains from higher levels of physical activity can promote a longer life with more independence and a higher quality of life. Physical activities, such as improving muscle strength and endurance, can also benefit older people who already have a physical disability. Older people do not have to engage in highly rigorous physical activity to prevent or reduce the risk of non-communicable diseases and falls. Moderate exercise, including walking and simple weight training, can be beneficial.

The potential impact of physical activities on health care expenditures is also significant. According to studies published by the Center for Diseases Control (CDC) in the United States, each dollar invested in physical activity (time and equipment) leads to $3.20 in medical cost saving. It is therefore no wonder that the US Surgeon General declared in his 1996 Report that "a sedentary lifestyle is hazardous to your health."

However, until the present time, much of the research on the positive impact of physical activities on how well we age has focused on populations in the developed work. Little is known about the long-term impact of the transition from physically active lifestyles in formerly agrarian societies in the developing world to modern urban life, characterised by increasing numbers of people working in hazardous conditions in jobs that may be high-stress, but require little or no physical activity. In spite of persistent poverty, their lives may be affected by changing nutritional patterns, such as fast food consumption, and other negative lifestyles, including smoking.

Research shows that both obesity and tobacco consumption are on the increase in developing countries. In developing and newly-industrialised countries, the burden of non-communicable diseases and injuries is expected to increase from 51 % to 78 % between 1990 and 2020. This increase is thought to be largely driven by population ageing, combined with exposure to tobacco and other risk factors, including physical inactivity. Furthermore, the urban environment in the new mega-cities of the developing world is often not conducive to recreational exercise because of crime rates, the lack of adequate recreational areas, such as public parks and sidewalks, and the rising rates of traffic accidents.

It is evident that the individual alone cannot be expected to be solely responsible for his or her health. At the policy-level, wide-ranging strategies are needed that create the economic, political and environmental conditions that promote health and support healthy behaviours. Promoting physical activities must go hand-in-hand with the recognition of a whole range of policy issues that touch such areas as urban planning, occupational safety and health, accident prevention and many others. This applies to both developing as well as developed countries.

Another area of concern, in both developed and particularly in developing countries, relates to culture and tradition and how they influence gender issues. Ageist and sexist attitudes in the developed world may pose difficulties for some older women to participate regularly in physical activities. For example, the sporting goods industry is only now beginning to catch on that many older women would enjoy opportunities for physical exercise, but do not necessarily enjoy putting on the tight leotards made for the 20-year old fitness enthusiast. Providing a safe and nurturing environment within which older women can engage in physical activities is of paramount importance for the success of such programmes. Similarly, culture and tradition in developing countries may make it difficult for women to walk, let alone exercise, in public. Gender-sensitive policies and programmes are necessary to ensure that all can benefit from activities and projects for better health. It is also important to promote a recognition of the benefits *for both men and women* of regular opportunities for physical activities, such as stair-climbing, housework, gardening, and last but certainly not least walking.

In 1999, during the International Year of Older Persons, WHO launched a global initiative highlighting the benefits of walking for older people. Under the banner of WHO's Global Embrace 1999, approximately one million older people and their families and friends in 97 countries celebrated and walked on the International Day of Older Persons in October 1999. Organisers in developing countries responded with particular enthusiasm as little attention had previously been given to health promotion for older people. New partnerships were forged on this occasion: service providers and medical centres linked with clubs and associations of older people, multisectoral NGO's linked with local government. Local partnerships for active ageing were key for planning the events.

The event was repeated this year on 1 October 2000 and it is hoped it will become a regular practice to celebrate it each year on the International Day of Older Persons. Professional associations, such as ICSSPE, are invited to join in and participate by publicising this event throughout their membership, publishing research results on the benefits of physical activities and ageing, and disseminating health messages through the WHO Global Embrace and as a partner in WHO's Global Movement for Active Ageing network.

New Perspectives on Sport History and Ageing

Patricia Vertinsky

Introduction

> "For the first time in history, most people can expect to
> live into the 'long late afternoon of life' ... [but] our
> culture is not much interested in why we grow old, how
> we ought to grow old or what it means to grow old ...
> [Perhaps] reweaving a collective past into the present,
> and reweaving a personal past into each stage of life
> are essential means of preparing for one's journey into
> the unknown future." (Cole, 1992:236, xxii, 250)

The value of a historical approach to ageing and sport is that it provides us with benchmarks against which we may measure current attitudes and approaches to the body, and poses models of past changes that may sensitise us to the forces transforming attitudes and structures in the present (Davison, 1995:59). Yet there are very few historical narratives of sport, exercise and ageing to illuminate the observations of French historian Georges Minois (1989:4) that "every society has the old people it deserves," and "each civilization has its model old person against which it judges all its old accordingly."

Even though the rapid ageing of Western society presses us to appreciate the health and exercise needs of ageing bodies, and acknowledge the role and benefits of sport across the life-span, you have to look very hard

Correspondence to: Prof. Dr. Patricia Vertinsky, Head, Department of Educational Studies, University of British Columbia, 2125 Main Mall, Vancouver, B.C., Canada, V6T 1Z4, Canada through the sport history journals to find studies of ageing sportsmen and women (Vertinsky and Cousins, 1999). While stories of old age experiences increasingly proliferate in libraries and bookstores we have not seen a corresponding spurt of historical interest in stories about elderly sport heroes, grandma's physical exploits or ageing fitness. It seems that until recently the thread of ageing has been largely overlooked, except through the popular biographies of (mostly male) retired athletes glorified in Halls of Fame, the occasional mention of local oldsters racing pigeons or cross country skiing, or prurient stories about the questionable management practices of personalities on international sporting committees who have held onto power well beyond middle age (Jennings, 1992; Kidd, 1997). From the sport historian's perspective the participation of elderly people in sport and exercise, as well as social and cultural attitudes toward the ageing body and its physical potential, remain relatively unexplored (Featherstone and Wernick, 1995; Vertinsky, 1998).

This is hardly surprising, since sport has been viewed so consistently in our culture as a young man's business - a history of male achievement and a celebration of youth, masculine strength, vigour and glory. In mainstream sport history at least, the historical study of sport has tended to focus upon the sporting pursuits of strong and able-bodied youth, to examine the wide variety of institutional arrangements in schools, clubs and colleges where their training in a variety of sports and physical education and exercise systems has taken place, and to trace their instrumental role in nation building, and imperial and colonial exploits. While many of us might agree that the body should be placed at the centre of all sporting discourse, it is nevertheless the youthful and vigorous, the machine-like albeit masculine body which remains the focus of most sporting historical narratives and which underlies the 'grand narrative' that encompasses the body's relation to sport.

As demographers point out, however, it is the ageing body which we now need to accommodate within this grand narrative. In 1800, only 2 % of the population was over 65 years of age; in 1900 over 4 % and by 1990 over 12 %. It is predicted to be 20 % by 2030. Today, older women over 65 years old outnumber men by 3 to 2, and over 85 by 3 to 1 (Golub, 1994). The ageing body, therefore, must be seen as one of the most important potential futures of the body and an inevitable one in light of increased longevity and the ageing of western society. As well, the 'feminisation' of ageing causes us to think carefully about the historical relationships between gender and sport. Feminists note that the invisible woman in history is the little old lady and that much of past and present writings about elderly subjects treat the male as the norm (Roebuck, 1985; Banner, 1993). They argue persuasively that a double standard of ageing has long existed for women, and that social and cultural factors have perpetuated the progressive discouragement of females from sport and physical activity as they age. What has made sport so uniquely effective as a medium for males is the case with which individuals have identified with the nation as symbolised by young persons - excelling at what practically every man wants to be good at (Hobsbawm, 1990). Thus the idealisation of a superior youthful body as an implicitly national symbol became a structural counterpart to the gendered female body of the invalid and dependant, and the relationship between weakness and gender slipped easily into a similar one with ageing, reinforcing common stereotypes of gender and age. If nations that idealise youthfulness and masculine strength stigmatise their old people what happens when we must confront the reality that age rather than youth is in the ascendancy? And, as ageing women multiply, what happens to that essence of an ideal citizen that has traditionally been reflected in the body of the male athlete or soldier's body? (Vertinsky, 1997).

In a rapidly ageing society we need to confront the possibility that emancipation from society's infatuation with youth could permit the choreographing of sport history in quite a new way (Vertinsky, 1998). Similarly we must revision mechanistic views of the body which have historically fostered negative rather than positive stereotypes and images about physically inactive elders and their deteriorating bodies. Our appreciation and criticism of sport will need to take cognisance of these historical determinants, and like other pioneering fields in social history, begin to confront the mass of popular and scholarly stereotypes that get in the way of a deeper understanding of the physical activities of ageing in the past and into the present (Blake, 1996).

We seize on myths because they help us make sense of life ... but we seize on them at a price, for the myths of ageing that we are fed in youth and middle age often provide an image of later life that is quite misleading and does not fit the typical experiences of older people (Thompson, Itzin and Abendstern, 1990; Bytheway et al., 1990).

Where, then, do we look to reconstruct a history of the ageing body, social attitudes toward elderly physicality, institutional arrangements for old people and the experiences of elders themselves at sport and play? In some respects the available literature is sparse, but we have not, perhaps, been looking in the right places, or hold too narrow a view of what sport and ageing have meant in times past. Fortunately, the current blossoming of histories of old age, theorising about the body (and its disciplining by institutions and the state), and a growing dialogue about the meaning and significance of later life, have begun to uncover new sources of information and shed new light upon the behaviour and treatment of the aged in the past. George Minois, Thomas Cole, Andrew Achenbaum, David Hackett Fischer, Peter Laslett, Carole Haber, and Stephen Katz, for example, have all provided scholarly examinations of ageing in the past and provided varying explanations (using different explanatory paradigms) for the elderly's position and behaviour in Western society. Perhaps the only consensus among the interesting works of these authors is that there is little agreement concerning when old age is supposed to begin, and that it is unlikely that there was ever a really a golden age for ageing - a time when ageing men and women were encouraged and supported to play appropriate sports and be as physically active as possible.

Achenbaum (1995) has argued that, although it is a fruitless distortion to invoke a single motif to capture the many and varied images of late life in Western society, bodily decline and disability have been dominant stereotypes leading to restrictions on the mobility and social and physical space of the elderly. For centuries, models of ageing represented bodies that grew and then steadily declined over the life course, becoming increasingly fixed and inflexible in terms of the cultural messages they were allowed to depict. From classical Greece until well beyond the Enlightenment, those who talked about appropriate behaviours for the elderly tended to view life from a life-course perspective, as a journey affected by contextual and personal factors, or saw it as a series of stages across the life course, like a staircase with predictable behaviours at each step (Burrow, 1986). At times these views existed simultaneously, supporting a spectrum of views about ageing physicality and the importance or inadvisability of exercise and sport, but the dominant tendency was to focus on old age as an inactive stage of life where sport had little role and passivity was the norm (Vertinsky, 1992). Females were typically perceived to age sooner than men; seen as sooner fit for reproduction, sooner mature for childbearing and sooner ready to wither in old age. Such beliefs contributed to the lasting notion that she should adopt passivity, inactivity and spectatorship earlier in life than her male counterpart (Vertinsky, 1995). What was important about these schemes of the stages of life was that they helped to provide the cognitive maps and behavioural norms for individuals to envision life as a natural sequence of roles and activities. Old people learned to acknowledge the limits of being old, not necessarily by how they felt, but by how they believed all old people should look and act, and, in the modern era, how the state came increasingly to insist upon it.

More optimistically, a number of historical studies of old age and exercise can be found in the fairly abundant literature on prolongevity, i.e., attempts to extend the lifespan through hygienic reforms such as diet, exercise and stress reduction. Among the more interesting recent studies to focus upon ageing and exercise are those of Peter Radford on eighteenth century pedestrians in England. Radford (1994, 1997) has collected fascinating data from old newspaper accounts about the exploits of aged male and female pedestrians and has analysed shifting public and medical attitudes toward physical exertion. His evidence suggests that most pedestrians were middle aged or old campaigners who walked or ran hundreds of miles across the country for wagers, and reported little trouble with extreme exertion into old age. "Mr. Eustace was 77 when he walked 216 miles in 1792, but the first prize for age and ability must go to Donald McLeod who was said to be 101 when he walked 1148 miles from Inverness to London and back" (Radford, 1997:5).

The historical literature on prolongevity has traditionally been used by kinesiologists in exploring attitudes toward exercise and ageing, though it has tended to obscure the complex role of class and the recreations of the common people in the study of ageing. Jack Berryman (1989) has explored the tradition of exercise and medicine from Hippocrates through ante-bellum America and Gerald Gruman (1961) has thoroughly documented the rise and fall of prolongevity hygiene. Of the numerous longevity treatises that became popular over the centuries, most are related to people of wealth and high birth, who, for a number of reasons (often dissipated lifestyles or ill health in youth) made strenuous efforts to live longer lives through moderating their lifestyles and incorporating exercise and sport. Again the standards of living, ageing and dying were conceptualised in male terms, with discussions of women invariably overdetermined by reference to female reproductive problems. Some examples of Renaissance work on bodily ageing include the writings of Gabriel Zerbi, an Italian physician who published Gerontocomia in 1489, a comprehensive review of forms of care for health and long life in old age. Unfortunately, before he could model his ideas on hygiene through his own long life, Zerbi was killed by the slaves of a Turkish pasha whose life he could not prolong (Demaitre, 1990). Louigi Cornaro was a sixteenth century Venetian nobleman who wrote *How to Live 100 Years and Avoid Disease* (1558), extolling personal hygiene and the simple life. Cornaro is said to have lived to 102 by following a daily diet of 12 ounces of bread, broth, egg yolks, and fresh meat together with 12 ounces of wine and by taking moderate exercise. His influential and optimistic work was widely distributed in Europe and America in the eighteenth and nineteenth centuries where it was generally seen as a health manual for ruling and common classes alike and was adopted by health reformers such as Sylvester Graham and Kellogg, of Kellogg's cornflakes (Gruman, 1966). In the spirit of these exemplars, many other writers from the seventeenth through the nineteenth centuries, such as George Cheyne's *An Essay on Health and Long Life* (1725) and Christopher Hufeland's *The Art of Prolonging Life* (1797), continued to discuss optimistic views on longevity and physical activity. Old age was certainly not seen to require specific medical attention until the early nineteenth century, when Sir John Sinclair's *Code of Health and Longevity* (1807) and Sir Andrew Carlisle's *An Essay on the Disorders of Old Age* (1817) began to recommend greater medical intervention in the lives of the elderly (Katz, 1996:30-40).

The emergence of the scientific and medical study of old age in the nineteenth century located disease as a necessary pathological condition of the elderly (Haber, 1983). Old age, which had earlier been regarded as a manifestation of the survival of the fittest, was removed from its ambiguous place in life's spiritual journey, and rationalised and redefined as a medical problem (Cole, 1992:xx). Nor was science served by the fact that many physicians, following Newtonian concepts of limited vital energy, believed that those who reached old age should try to conserve the last remnants of the finite portion of energy allotted to the life-span by severely limiting physical effort. Ageing became likened to a worn-out and degenerating body-machine - an affliction for which there seemed to be few remedies. In spite of a continuing tradition by prolongevity experts, the decline in the status of the elderly grew steadily worse during the nineteenth century as the medical profession exacerbated negative attitudes toward old age as a period of weakness and obsolescence requiring cautious age- and gender-appropriate behaviour. Over-exertion was sternly warned against for it might easily lead to cardiac arrest and a host of life threatening conditions. Most significant was the application and acceptance of conservative prescriptions for exercise at a much earlier age for women than men, socialising the former, while still in their 40's, to take on sedentary characteristics of ageing by disengaging from active pursuits and anxiously conserving their body machine.

Where sport and exercise were concerned, the notion of ageing as a disease and period of inevitable decline and dependency requiring professional help and medical techniques had lasting and often damaging consequences. To be sure, we can find occasional stories of the marvellous exploits of active elderly folk and the sporting pursuits of the rich and famous at a mature age, but when we examine the popular journals and the medical literature of the late nineteenth century and well into the twentieth, we are struck by the cautionary and repressive advice to ageing men and women (especially women) to restrict their physicality and 'act their age' (Vertinsky, 1991, 1992). Thus science, medicine, social Darwinism and accelerated industrialisation lead to what has been labelled a watershed in the history of old age.

"An emerging scrap heap of older industrial workers, the medical recognition of old age as a clinically distinct period of life, and the early stages of an epidemiological transition from infectious to degenerative diseases, all drew attention to decay, dependency, and pathology in old age" (Cole, 1983:37). Currently, there are a number of useful efforts to revise gerontological histories - to undiscipline old age, as Stephen Katz (1996) puts it, and to look more closely at the modernisation thesis held rather firmly by gerontologists until recently. Cultural studies, social and cultural historians, human geographers, sociologists and medical anthropologists have entered the field of ageing and are looking critically at the social construction of ageing and the ageing body (Chudacoff, 1989). Although critics have bemoaned gerontology's relative immunity to the fresh breezes of postmodernism, feminism, semiotics and other theoretical approaches, there is exciting new work developing in these areas. Golden age historical stereotypes have been deconstructed and debunked, and images and representations of old age in literature, art, poetry and at work, sport and play are increasingly being explored. Postmodernists such as Mike Featherstone and Andrew Wernick (1995) are examining representational discourses and images, blurring chronological boundaries and pressing for the integration of formerly segregated periods of life. It is increasingly understood that the ageing body (however that is constructed) is part of the domain of history, culture and meaning, and not - as medicine would have it - an ahistorical, pre-social, purely natural object. Indeed, through the new lexicon of postmodernity, the ageing body has stolen into the spotlight as something to grasp, something that has a history in an increasingly somatic society. "Old age is no longer, if it ever was, the mellow withdrawal from life's contradictions and possibilities it was thought to be" (Katz, 1996:7). New modes of inquiry, new paradigms through which we can explore the ageing body, more sophisticated understandings of power and gender/age relations, and the pressure of growing numbers of active old people upon sporting and recreational institutions, public space and public policy, all combine to make ageing an essential and potentially fruitful focus for sport historians.

The old adage that 'you've reached old age when all you exercise is caution' is no longer proving to be true of ageing men and women, their exercise habits and their sporting displays. Sport historians are beginning to portray the agency of ageing individuals at sport and illustrate how growing old cannot be understood apart from its subjective experience, mediated by social condition and cultural significance. Today's history can be rethought as microhistory, locality, autobiography, even anecdotal history, as a recent article on sport veterans in Finland nicely shows. Here the informal relating of what once might have been thought of as "small and trivial things," through interviews with sport veterans and the discovery of old photographs, medals, clippings and home videos, has encouraged the development of a new kind of living museum of sports for local communities to display at sites where those sports are still practised and watched. In the local sites where large crowds spend time watching and playing, oral traditions are circulated and memories rekindled through displays and media shows. Through such methods, it is suggested sport 'spaces' can become sport 'places' once again - meaningful sites with their own traditions and identities - places with a history of sport (Sironen, Karkkainen and Silvennoinen, 1997).

References

Achenbaum, W.A. (1978). *Old age in the new land: The American experience since 1790*. Baltimore: Johns Hopkins University Press.

Banner, L.W. (1993). *In full flower: Ageing women, power and sexuality*. New York: Vintage Books.

Berryman, J.W. (1989). The tradition of the 'six-things non-natural': Exercise and medicine from Hippocrates through ante-bellum America. *Exercise and Sport Sciences Review*, 17, 515-559.

Blake, A. (1996). *The body language: The meaning of modern sport*. London: Lawrence and Wishart.

Burrow, J.A. (1986). *The ages of man: A study in medieval writing and thought*. Oxford: Clarendon Press.

Bytheway, B., Keil, T., Allatt, P., & Bryman, A. (Eds.) (1990*). Becoming and being old. Sociological approaches to later life*. London: Sage.

Chudacoff, H. (1989). *How old are you? Age consciousness in American culture*. Princeton: Princeton University Press.

Cole, T.R. (1983, June). *The enlightened view of ageing: Victorian morality in a new key*. The Hastings Center Report.

Davison, G. (1995). Our youth is spent and our backs are bent: The origins of Australian ageism. *Australian Cultural History*, 14, 40-62.

Demaitre, L. (1990). The care and extension of old age in medieval medicine. In M.M. Sheehan (Ed.), *Ageing and the aged in medieval Europe* (pp. 3-22). Toronto: Pontifical Institute of Medieval Studies.

Golub, E.S. (1994). *The limits of medicine*. New York: Random House.

Gruman, G.T. (1961). The rise and fall of prolongevity hygiene, 1558-1873. *Bulletin of the History of Medicine*, 35, 221-229.

Haber, C. (1983). *Beyond sixty-five. The dilemma of old age in America's past*. Cambridge: Cambridge University Press.

Hobsbawn, E. (1990). *Nations and nationalism since 1780. Programme, myth, reality*. Cambridge: Cambridge University Press.

Jennings, A. (1992). *The Lord of the Rings: Power, money and drugs in the modern Olympics*. Toronto: Stoddart.

Kerzer, D.I., and Laslett, P. (Eds.) (1995). *Ageing in the past: Demography, society and old age*. Berkeley, CA: University of California Press.

Kidd, B. (1997). Missing: Women from sports halls of fame. In P. Donnelly (Ed.), *Taking sport seriously: Social issues in Canadian sports* (pp. 311-313). Toronto: Thompson Educational Pub. Inc.

Minois, G. (1989). *A history of old age: From Antiquity to the Renaissance*. Trans. Sarah Hanbury Tenison. Chicago: Chicago University Press.

Radford, P. (1997, July). *Escaping the Philippedes connection: Death and illness in 18th century sport in Britain*. Paper presented at the IVth Congress of the International Society for the History of Physical Education and Sport: Lyon.

Radford, P. (1994). Women's foot races in the 18th and 19th centuries. A popular and widespread practice. *Canadian Journal of History of Sport*, 25, 1, 57-68.

Roebuck, J. (1985). *The invisible woman is a little old lady: The need for change in assumptions and paradigms*. Paper presented at the annual meeting of the Gerontological Society of America: San Antonio, Texas.

Sironen, E., Kärkkäinen, P., & Silvennoinen, M. (1997, November). On narrative locality in sports: An experiment. *The Sports Historian*, 17, 2, 44-53.

Troyansky, D.G. (1989). *Old age in the old regime*. Ithaca: Cornell University Press.

Vertinsky, P. (1998, May). Ageing bodies, ageing sport historians and the choreographing of sport history. *Sport History Review*, 19, 1, 18-29.

Vertinsky, P. (1997, July). *Fitness narratives: The medicalization and gendering of the ageing body and physical body*. Paper presented at the IVth Congress of the International Society for the History of Physical Education and Sport: Lyon.

Vertinsky, P. (1992). Sport and exercise for old women: Images of the elderly in the medical and popular literature at the turn of the century. *International Journal of the History of Sport*, 9, 1, 83-104.

Non-Specialist Bibliography

Achenbaum, A.W. (1995). Images of old age in America, 1790-1970. A vision and revision. In M. Featherstone and A. Wernick (Eds.), *Images of aging* (pp. 19-28).

Cole, T.R. (1992). *The journey of life: A cultural history of aging in America*. Cambridge: Cambridge University Press.

Featherstone, M., & Wernick. A. (1995). *Images of aging: Cultural representations of later life*. London: Routledge.

Fischer, D.H. (1978). *Growing old in America*. Oxford: Oxford University Press.

Katz, S. (1996). *Disciplining old age. The formation of gerontological knowledge*. Charlottsville and London: University Press of Virginia.

Laslett, P. (1990). *A fresh map of life: The emergence of the third age*. London: Weidenfeld and Nicolson.

Thompson, P., Itzin, C., & Abendstern, M. (1990). *I don't feel old. The experience of late life*. Oxford: Oxford University Press.

Vertinsky, P., & O'Brien Cousins, S. (1999, forthcoming). Aging, gender and physical activity. In K. Young and P. White (Eds.), *Sport and gender in Canada*. Oxford: Oxford University Press.

Vertinsky, P. (1995). Stereotypes of aging women and exercise: An historical perspective. *Journal of Aging and Physical Activity*, 3, 3, 223-238.

Vertinsky, P. (1991). Old age, gender and physical activity. The biomedicalization of aging. *Journal of Sport History*, 18, 2.

The Role of Physical Activity in the Prevention of Osteoporosis: The Importance of Starting Young

Donald A. Bailey

Introduction

Recent evidence suggesting an increase in the incidence and prevalence of osteoporosis (WHO, 1994) has renewed interest in lifestyle factors, in particular weight-bearing physical activity and dietary calcium as potential contributors in the prevention of this chronic condition. Although osteoporosis is primarily a disease of older adults, the failure to attain an optimum level of bone mineral during the years of growth is likely to be a significant contributing cause of dangerously low bone mineral conditions in older populations (Bailey & McCulloch, 1992). The inverse relationship between bone mineral status and fracture risk has been well documented to the point where the World Health Organization, for the purposes of diagnosis, defines osteoporosis as bone mineral 2.5 standard deviations (SD) below the mean for bone mineral in young adults (WHO, 1994).

While heredity is a major determinant of bone mineral status, a recent study indicates that nearly one-half the variance in bone mineral can be attributed to non-hereditary factors (Krall & Dawson-Hughes, 1993) and there is evidence that physical activity may be an important contributing factor. Within genetic limits, vigorous weight-bearing physical activity and adequate calcium intake represent the best possibility for enhancing the attainment of an optimum level of bone mineral.

Correspondence to: Prof. Dr. D.A. Bailey, College of Kinesiology, University of Saskatchewan, 105 Gymnasium Place, Saskatoon, SK, S7N 5C2, Canada
Additional Affiliation and Address: Department of Human Movement Studies, University of Queensland, Brisbane, Qld. 4072, Australia.

Bone Mineral Acquisition During Growth

Our understanding of osteoporosis in the elderly is limited by our lack of knowledge concerning the determinants of bone mineral acquisition during the years of growth. Adult bone mineral status is a reflection of bone mineral accrual during growth and subsequent loss with advancing years. The establishment of an optimum level of bone mineral in childhood and adolescence is of crucial concern in terms of lifelong skeletal adequacy. Because bone mineral loss is a normal consequence of ageing, those who acquire a greater bone mineral balance during the first two decades of life should be at reduced risk for the health problems associated with skeletal fragility later in life.

To explore the possibility of optimising bone mineral acquisition during the years of growth and gain an understanding of modifiable factors that may promote skeletal health, it is first necessary to have an understanding of typical bone mineral accrual rates in normal growing children. To investigate how bone mineral is laid down at clinically important sites during the adolescent years, data from an initial sample of 228 children measured annually by dual energy X-ray absorptiometry (DXA) over a six year period were analysed (Bailey, 1997). To address maturational differences between boys and girls of the same chronological age, bone mineral content (BMC) values were determined at points two years on either side of the age of peak height velocity (PHV) which was used as a benchmark of maturity. The results of this study indicate that in the four years surrounding PHV, 35 % of total body and lumbar spine BMC is laid down, and 27 % of femoral neck BMC is accumulated. These values are in agreement with a study by Slemenda et al. (1994), who reported a 29 % increase in BMC at the lumbar spine in the three years around the onset of puberty. The clinical significance of these findings can best be appreciated by considering the fact that as much bone mineral will be laid down during the four adolescent years surrounding PHV as many people will lose during their entire adult life.

Another issue of clinical significance has to do with the observation that during adolescence there is a dissociation between linear growth and bone mineral accrual (Bailey, Faulkner & McKay, 1996). For all bone sites in both boys and girls, peak velocity in BMC occurs up to one year after PHV.

This suggests a transient period of relative bone weakness following the adolescent growth spurt, resulting in a temporary increase in fracture risk. The relationship between fracture incidence in children and the timing of the adolescent growth spurt has been well documented, with fracture rates increasing dramatically during the circumpubertal years. (Alffram & Bauer, 1962; Bailey et al., 1989; Blimkie et al., 1993). This research further emphasises the importance of studying the dynamics of bone mineral changes during the years of growth.

The observation that adolescence is a critical time for bone mineral accumulation should not be surprising. By the time growth ceases, the skeleton should be as strong as it will ever need to be (Parfitt, 1994). Gains in bone mineral after growth has ceased are probably minimal (Slemendra et al., 1994). Since 50 % of the variability in bone mass in the very old can be accounted for by peak skeletal mass attained during the growing years (Hui, Johnston & Mazess, 1985), it is not unreasonable to assume that fracture risk in the elderly may have childhood antecedents (Bailey & McCulloch, 1992). Clearly, more information is needed regarding the precise relationship between modifiable lifestyle factors like physical activity and nutritional intake and bone mineral accumulation during the growing years.

Bone Mineral Acquisition and Physical Activity

Two recent reviews provide a detailed discussion of childhood and adolescent physical activity in relation to bone mineral (Bailey, Faulkner & McKay, 1996; Barr & McKay, 1998). The authors of these reviews concluded that the available evidence was strongly supportive, suggesting a positive relationship between physical activity and bone mineral accrual. There was, however, some degree of inconsistency in the results. This could be attributed, in part, to limitations in study design. These included small numbers of subjects, lack of control and short duration of exercise interventions, the difficulty in accurately assessing physical activity patterns in children and adolescents, and the failure to control for maturational differences during adolescence.

Preferred limb studies provide some of the most convincing evidence as to the positive effects of physical activity. These unilateral control studies provide an excellent experimental model for studying the effect of mechanical loading on bone mineral acquisition. Because genetic, endocrine and nutritional influences are shared by both limbs, any bilateral disparity in bone mineral accumulation can safely be attributed to differences in mechanical usage.

One such study of 105 elite young adult (18-28 yr.) female tennis and squash players provides an excellent illustration of the effects of childhood physical activity on bone (Kannus et al., 1995). The bilateral difference in bone mineral content between the playing and non-playing arms was measured and compared to similar determinations on 50 healthy control subjects of similar age, height and weight. Although the controls had approximately 4 % higher bone mineral content in the dominant over the non-dominant humerus (attributed to activities of daily living), the young athletes who began playing and training for their sport at or before menarche had bilateral differences of 17-24 %. Those who began training after menarche had differences of 8-14 %. Clearly, the greater bone mineral in the playing arm reflects the strains imposed on this limb by the sport. The starting age appears to be an important consideration, emphasising the greater adaptive response to loading in immature bone over mature bone (Forwood & Burr, 1993).

In another preferred limb study, bone mineral density (BMD) was measured by DXA in regions of the involved and non-involved proximal femur in 17 children (7-14 yr.) with unilateral Legg Calve Perthes Disease (Bailey et al., 1997). Children with this condition have an altered weight-bearing pattern whereby there is increased mechanical loading on the non-involved normal hip and reduced loading on the involved painful hip. Thus, these children provide a unique opportunity to study the impact of differential loading on bone mineral acquisition during the growing years while controlling for genetic and other factors. A significantly higher BMD was found for regions of the proximal femur on the non-involved side over the involved side (4 to 15 %) and regions on the non-involved side were significantly greater than either chronological or skeletal age based norms. The results of this study provide further support for the concept that mechanical loading of the skeleton during the growing years is an important factor in bone mineral acquisition.

Recent studies have provided further evidence indicating that physical activity during youth is associated with a higher bone mineral status (Boot et al., 1997; Cassell, Benedict & Specker, 1996; Dyson et al., 1997; Gunnes & Lehman, 1996). In one of the few prospective studies on young children, 38 girls (9-10 yr.) were enrolled in an additional exercise program over and above their regular physical education classes (Morris et al., 1997). The extra classes of 30 minutes duration were held three times per week for ten months and involved high impact-loading and strength-building exercises. At the end of the study period, gains in BMC were compared to a control group of 33 girls who had participated only in the regular physical education classes. Bone mineral content for the total body, proximal femur and lumbar spine increased at a significantly greater rate in the exercise group compared with the controls (7 to 12 % vs 1.5 to 6 %). These results suggest that high-impact exercise is beneficial in terms of bone mineral acquisition in children. More importantly, this study indicates that carefully planned exercise programmes can be designed to fulfil the goal of increasing the bone mineral status in children as part of the school curriculum.

In a longitudinal study of normal children, 60 boys and 53 girls were measured annually over a 6-year period. Bone mineral accrual rates at the lumbar spine, femoral neck and total body were found to be significantly related to physical activity patterns as measured by multiple questionnaire assessments taken each year (Bailey et al., 1996). To control for the well documented maturational differences between children of the same chronological age, comparisons between children in different activity groups were made at similar developmental ages (age of peak accrual plus 1 year and minus 1 year) as opposed to chronological age comparisons. To control for size differences, height and weight were entered as covariates in the statistical analyses. After controlling for maturational and size differences between activity groups, active children accumulated significantly more bone mineral in the 2 year period around peak than their inactive peers. These findings in favour of the active children were consistent across all sites. This study is unique in demonstrating that bone mineral accrual rates across the adolescent years are dependent on the level of normal everyday physical activity.

Studies that have investigated the response of growing bone in young animals have been reviewed by Forwood and Burr (1993). As a result of this review, these investigators concluded that the animal studies provide incontrovertible evidence that growing bone has a greater capacity to add new bone to the skeleton in response to mechanical loading factors than mature bone. The consistency of the evidence suggests that the animal data have relevance for humans. Considered as a whole, the studies noted above and the animal and human review papers suggest that bone mineral in children can be enhanced by loading factors associated with physical activity.

Conclusion

The differential effect of loading on the growing skeleton as opposed to the mature skeleton supports the contention that adequate physical activity during the growing years is more important for increasing bone mineral than exercise undertaken later in life (Forwood & Burr, 1993). There is strong support for participation in weight-bearing physical activity to optimise bone mineral acquisition early in life and maintain it through exercise during the adult years. The primary benefit of physical activity in the elderly is in the reduction of age-related bone loss and the improvement in aspects of fitness, particularly strength, flexibility and balance which may help to prevent falls and the associated risk of fractures.

While there are still more questions than answers, clearly, studies of osteoporosis are needed that address not only age-related bone loss, but also bone gain during the growing years. The ultimate target population for the prevention of osteoporosis may be the young and not the elderly (Chestnut, 1991). Taking into account the fact that our knowledge of the complicated mechanisms controlling bone mineral status is still incomplete, on the basis of what we do know it is possible to offer some sound and prudent lifestyle advice to young people.

With regard to exercise programmes designed for skeletal health and bone acquisition in the young, the following fundamentals should be kept in mind; a) exercise programs do not elicit benefits that can be generalised to the whole skeleton, b) the skeletal response to exercise is greatest at the site of maximum stress and c) to effect an adaptive response, the training stimulus must be greater than that habitually encountered. On the basis of these fundamentals and the review of the pertinent literature the following recommendations can safely be offered to the public at large.

1. An individual should make a lifelong commitment to physical activity at an early age. Growing bones respond to weight-bearing activity by the addition of new bone. The ability to adapt to increases in mechanical loading is much greater in the growing skeleton than in the mature skeleton.
2. Weight-bearing activities that provide impact loading like gymnastics, skipping, aerobics, squash, basketball etc. are better for the skeleton than weight-supported activities such as swimming or cycling.
3. A variety of vigorous daily activities of short duration which provide a versatile strain distribution throughout the entire skeleton is better for bone health than a prolonged repetitive activity.
4. Activities should be diverse to ensure a varied strain distribution on bone, they should be vigorous enough to ensure impact loading with high strain rates, and they should be progressive in nature.
5. Activities that increase muscle strength and work all large muscle groups should be encouraged as these can be osteogenic, however, static loads applied continuously are not in and of themselves osteogenic.
6. As much as possible, periods of immobility and immobilisation should be avoided; when this is not possible because of sickness or injury, even brief periods of daily weight-bearing movements can help to conserve bone mineral. The responsiveness of the growing skeleton to physical activity is dependent on the sensitivity of bone to circulating hormone levels and nutritional adequacy. This has important implications for exercise prescription in adolescents which leads to a number of other important recommendations.
7. Children should have a diet of nutritious foods that will meet the recommended dietary intake for calcium, provide adequate but not excessive protein and limit the intake of sodium and caffeinated beverages (soft drinks, coffee).
8. In girls, abnormal delay of menarche and menstrual dysfunction, associated with a chronic energy deficit, represents a potential skeletal hazard in terms of bone mineral acquisition and maintenance. A well-balanced diet that is sufficient to meet the energy demands of

growth and physical activity should be encouraged. This will facilitate the onset and maintenance of a normal menstrual cycle.

9. Disordered eating habits are destructive to the skeleton at any age; when this occurs during the growing years there may be a permanent deficit in bone mineral status throughout life.

10. Cigarettes should be avoided; they are anti-estrogenic and may interfere with the attainment of an optimum level of bone mineral following skeletal maturation.

References
(* denotes references which would be of particular interest to non-specialists)

Alffram, P.A. & Bauer, G.C.H. (1962). Epidemiology of fractures of the forearm. *Journal of Bone and Joint Surgery*, 44, 105-114. 1962.

Bailey, D.A. & McCulloch, R.G. (1992). Osteoporosis: are there childhood antecedents for an adult health problem? *Canadian Journal of Pediatrics*, 5, 130-134.

Bailey, D.A., Wedge, J.H., McCulloch, R.G., Martin, A.D., & Bernhardson, S.C. (1989). Epidemiology of fractures of the distal end of the radius in children as associated with growth. *Journal of Bone and Joint Surgery*, 71, 1225-1231.

Bailey, D.A., Faulkner, R.A., Kimber, K., Dzus, A. & Yong-Hing, K. (1997). Altered loading patterns and femoral bone mineral density in children with unilateral legg-calvé-perthes disease. *Medicine and Science in Sports and Exercise*, 29, 1395-1399.

*Bailey, D.A. (1997). The Saskatchewan pediatric bone mineral accrual study: bone mineral acquisition during the growing years. *International Journal of Sports Medicine*, 18, (S3), 191-194.

*Bailey, D.A., McKay, H.A., Mirwald, R.L., Crocker, P.E. & Faulkner, R.A. (1999). A six-year longitudinal study of the relationship of physical activity to bone mineral accrual in growing children: The University of Saskatchewan Bone Mineral Accrual Study. *Journal of Bone and Mineral Research,* 14, 1672-1679.

*Bailey, D.A., Faulkner, R.A. & McKay, H.A. (1996). Growth, physical activity and bone mineral acquisition. In *Exercise and Sport Sciences Reviews*, volume 24, J.O. Holloszy (Ed.). Baltimore: Williams and Wilkins, pp. 122-166.

*Barr, S.I. & McKay, H.A. (1998). Nutrition, exercise and bone status in youth. *International Journal of Sport Nutrition*, 8(2), 24-142.

Blimkie, C.J.R., Levevre, J., Beunen, G.P., Renson, R. Dequeker, J. & Van Damme, P. (1993). Fractures, physical activity, and growth velocity in adolescent Belgian boys. *Medicine and Science in Sports and Exercise*, 25, 801-808.

Boot, A.M., de Ridder, M.A.J., Pols, H.A.P., Krenning, E.P. & de Muinck Keizer-Schrama, S.M.P.F. (1997). Bone mineral density in children and adolescents: relation to puberty, calcium intake and physical activity. *Journal of Clinical Endocrinology and Metabolism,* 82,57-62.

Cassell, C., Benedict, M. & Specker, B. (1996). Bone mineral density in elite 7-9 year-old female gymnasts and swimmers. *Medicine and Science in Sports and Exercise*, 28, 1243-1246.

Chestnut, C. (1991). Theoretical overview: bone development, peak bone mass, bone loss, and fracture risk. *American Journal of Medicine*, 91(53), 2S-4S.

Dyson, K., Blimkie, C.J.R., Davison, K.S., Webber, C.E. & Adachi, J.D. (1997). Gymnastics training and bone density in pre-adolescent females *Medicine and Science in Sports and Exercise*, 29, 443-450.

Forwood, M. & Burr, D. (1993). Physical activity and bone mass: exercise in futility? *Bone Mineral*, 21, 89-112.

Gunnes, M. & Lehman E. (1996). Physical activity and dietary constituents as predictors of forearm cortical and trabecular bone gain in healthy children and adolescents: a prospective study. *Acta Paediatrics*, 85, 19-25.

Hui, S.L., Johnston, C.C. & Mazess, R.B. (1985). Bone mass in normal children and young adults. *Growth*, 49, 34-43.

Kannus, P., Haapasalo, H., Sankelo, M., Sievanen, H., Pasanen, M., Heinonen, A., Oja, P. & Vuori, I. (1995). Effect of starting age of physical activity on bone mass in the dominant arm of tennis and squash players. *Annals of Internal Medicine,* 123, 27-31.

Krall, E., & Dawson-Hughes, B. (1993). Heritable and lifestyle determinants of bone mineral density. *Journal of Bone and Mineral Research*, 8, 1-9.

Morris, F., Naughton, G., Gibbs, J., Carlson, J. & Wark, J. (1997). Prospective 10-month exercise intervention in pre-menarcheal girls: positive effects on bone and lean mass. *Journal of Bone and Mineral Research*, 12, 1453-1462.

Parfitt, A.M. (1994). The two faces of growth: benefits and risks to bone integrity. *Osteoporosis International*, 4, 382-398.

Slemenda, C.W., Reister, T.K., Hui, S.L., Miller, J.Z., Christian, J.C. & Johnston, C.C. (1994). Influences on skeletal mineralization in children and adolescents: Evidence for varying effects of sexual maturation and physical activity. *Journal of Pediatrics*, 125, 201-207.

World Health Organization. (1994). Assessment of fracture risk and its application to screening for postmenopausal osteoporosis. *Report of WHO Study Group*, WHO, Geneva.

Exercise and Training in Ageing

Michael Sagiv

Work capacity

The ageing influence on work capacity and physical performance and during exercise has been widely investigated. It has been found that there are changes in the heart, lung and skeletal muscles which reduce physical performance with advancing age (Conway, Wheeler & Sannerstedt, 1971; Sagiv et al., 1986). Myocardial functional changes with ageing in sedentary adults include a decline in maximal heart rate, stroke volume, and contractility, and an increase in peripheral vascular resistance. The changes in structure and function of the cardiovascular system result in a decline in maximal oxygen uptake (VO2max), which is the best single indicator of physical working capacity. Whether maximal cardiac output actually decreases with primary ageing depends on many interactive factors. First, the primary ageing process, which has a genetic component, occurs in the absence of disease and independent of life-style (Hoeldtke & Cilms, 1985). If oxygen transport is indeed limited by maximal cardiac output, this may be calculated as the product of maximal heart rate, arterio-venous oxygen difference, and maximal stroke volume.

The second possible cause that may reduce VO2max with ageing is the reduced arterio-venous oxygen difference at maximal effort (Shephard, 1987). The elderly are not generally anemic and the red blood cell content is usually well maintained, although it may decrease in subjects with a large VO2max (Dempsey, 1987). Some studies have shown correlation between

Correspondence to: Prof. Dr. Michael Sagiv, Zinman College of Physical Education, Wingate Institute, Wingate Post Office, 42902, Israel

VO2max and muscle mass (Fleg & Lakatta, 1988; Rodgers et al., 1990). Mitochondrial density was found to be lower in skeletal muscle of older individuals, which could further diminish capacity for endurance work. Thus, it may be that the ageing-related atrophy of skeletal muscle plays some role in the ageing-related decline in work endurance (Booth, Weeden & Tseng, 1994; Kallinen et al., 1998).

However, other studies (Hagberg et al., 1989; Pollock et al., 1987) do not support a causal role for muscular atrophy in the decline in VO2max during ageing. It seems that the related changes in VO2max are dependent on a number of factors including the onset of disease and level of physical activity. The lowest rates of decline in VO2max with age are found in those who remain disease-free and continue to maintain high levels of physical activity. Over a 10-year period, no significant decline in VO2max was found in a group of competitive masters athletes who maintained their training intensity and continued to compete. The annual rate of decay in VO2max for the general population is estimated to be: 0.4–0.5ml $\cdot$ kg$^{-1} \cdot$ min$^{-1} \cdot$ year^{-1}. The highest rates of decline in VO2max are in those individuals who have reduced their levels of physical activity as they age.

Cardiopulmonary changes

Changes in the structure of the cardiopulmonary system appear to be influenced by age, disease and the level of physical activity. Some changes appear to occur independent of gender, disease and level of physical activity. Other structural changes, such as an increase in the left ventricular mass, appear to be dependent on both gender and the level of physical activity.

In the cardiovascular system, morphological and physiological changes have been identified in the elderly. The morphological changes typically do not produce clinical signs of cardiac dysfunction during life. In the elderly, there is a modest increase in left ventricular thickness, probably resulting from the observed increase in systolic blood pressure. Except for increased tortuosity, cross-sectional area, and degree of atherosclerosis, there are no clear age-associated changes in coronary arteries. However, studies in this area are limited.

Ageing is associated with a shift in the mechanism by which cardiac output is maintained during submaximal exercise. In spite of the elderly having a lower early diastolic filling rate during submaximal exercise, end-diastolic volume (the amount of blood filled in the ventricle at the end of diastole) is maintained and even increased as a function of age. As a result, older subjects appear to have a greater reliance on the Frank-Starling mechanism for the maintenance of cardiac output during submaximal exercise. The decrease of maximal heart rate associated with advanced age is similar for the sedentary person, the average active person and the top athlete. In humans, maximal heart rate peaks at around 10 years of age and decreases by approximately 1 beat $\cdot$ min^{-1} $\cdot$ year^{-1}. This suggests that maximal heart rate does not adapt to chronic exercise (Ehsani et al., 1991). The mechanism(s) underlying the decreased maximal heart rate is unknown. The changes may be attributed to the heart itself rather than to neural input. An example for the input ability of the nervous system in the elderly is the manifestation of ventricular arrhythmias. Ventricular tachycardia at a rate of 200 beat $\cdot$ min^{-1} is observed in elderly persons who could not attain this heart rate by physiological means (Tate, Hyek & Taffet, 1994). Moreover, changes in the number of pacemaker cells and volume of the sinoatrial node result from ageing (Capasso et al., 1989). Other investigations suggested that there is an age-related decline in maximal heart rate which could be associated with decreased sympathetic drive (Lakatta, 1993), due to diminished response to adrenergic regulation of the heart and circulation (Bertel et al., 1980).

Older subjects rely on changes in stroke volume by dilatation of the left ventricle during intermediate and maximal exercise to partially maintain cardiac output and to compensate for the reduction in heart rate (Sagiv et al., 1989). However, maximal stroke volume is decreased due to reduced preload (circulating blood volume associated with physical inactivity) and increased afterload. Thus, the perfusion of the working muscles via many regulatory mechanisms is reduced. Age appears to be associated with an increase in the total peripheral resistance independent of change in maximal limb blood flow, however, studies suggest that age is associated with a decrease in the maximal conductance of the vascular bed of the calf. Endurance training results in an increase in the maximal conductance independent of age, but the mechanism for the change in maximal limb conduction with age is not well understood. At peak exercise, older individuals tend to show a greater increase in end-diastolic volume and end-systolic volume when compared with younger subjects (Rodeheffer et al., 1984). The changes in left ventricular volume during exercise may be due to reduced contractility, diastolic and systolic left ventricular functions and loading conditions. The failure to augment contractility in the older subjects may be the cause of reduced diastolic and systolic functions.

Contractility appears diminished with age. Compared to the young, older subjects have a greater end-systolic volume and a lower ejection fraction during submaximal exercise. The mechanism(s) for the decrease in contractility with age are unclear, however, increased afterload, and/or a decreased responsiveness to adrenergic stimulation have been suggested.

Maximal isometric contractile properties of left ventricular muscle are altered in old humans (Tate, Hyek & Taffet, 1994). The contraction duration is prolonged and may result from a decrease in the rate of calcium transport by cardiac sarcoplasmic reticulum (Tate et al., 1990). Similarly, the isotonic contractile properties are altered with ageing (Capasso et al., 1989), leading to changes in two variables of isotonic contraction: velocity of shortening and relaxation time. These changes in isometrically and isotonically contracting cardiac muscle (shown in isolated cardiac muscle from rats) lower peak filling of the heart of elderly humans. Recently, diastolic left ventricular filling has been shown to be affected not only by ventricular property, but also by ageing (Downes et al., 1989; Kuo et al., 1987). Therefore, ageing is associated with a shift of left ventricular filling from early to late, decreasing the passive/active phases of filling ratio diastole. Thus, the heart relies more on atrial filling, and an increase in isovolumic relaxation time indicating diastolic dysfunction (Sagiv, Goldhammer & Ben-Sira, 1992).

Left ventricular systolic performance is well-maintained with ageing under resting conditions. However, systolic function is reduced during exercise. This response may be mediated, at least in part, by age-associated reductions in beta-adrenergic receptor sensitivity or density, reducing the inotropic response of the myocytes to a standard dose of catecholamine (Shephard, 1989). Another manifestation of the decreased responsiveness of cardiovascular tissues to beta-adrenergic stimulation is the decreased ability of the atrium to dilate. The peripheral vasculature, however, does not show decreased vasodilatation by the vasodilatating stimuli of nitrates, indicating that the vascular changes are receptor-mediated rather than intrinsic (Weisfeldt & Gerstenblith, 1986). Thus, blood pressure and mean systemic blood pressure increase progressively with age, both at rest and during exercise. This rise in total peripheral resistance may affect left ventricular loading conditions, which in turn may mask or mimic changes in left ventricular volumes, diastolic and systolic functions (Gardin et al., 1987; Stoddard et al., 1989).

Numerous structural and functional changes in the lung, chest wall respiratory muscles, and vasculature occur with age (Krumpe et al., 1985; Levitzky, 1984). Four major changes appear to affect lung function, pulmonary mechanics, and respiratory flow rates as ageing occurs. The primary change is a decrease in elastic recoil of the lung tissue (Islam, 1980), and to a lesser extent a stiffening of the chest wall due to a decrease in intervertebral space (Mauderly & Hahn, 1982) and an apparent loss of respiratory muscle strength (Black & Hyatt, 1969). These result in a reduction of arterial oxygen partial pressure, maximal voluntary ventilation, force expiratory volumes, total lung capacity, vital capacity and pulmonary diffusing capacity, and increases in functional residual capacity, residual volume, physiological dead space and time required for mixing inhaled air (Johnson et al., 1991a; Johnson et al., 1991b; Johnson & Dempsey, 1991).

Muscle and energy system

Metabolism is the sum of all the chemical reactions that occur within the body. ATP is essential for all physiological functions because it provides energy. Therefore, muscle contraction is dependent on a supply of ATP, which is presented in a low concentration within the muscle (5 mmol . kg^{-1} wet muscle) and has to be resynthesised from ADP by two major pathways, namely, anaerobic and aerobic. Although these two processes, anaerobic and aerobic, are described separately for convenience, they are invariable in dynamic equilibrium and their relative contribution to NAD resynthesis depends on the availability of oxygen. Thus, muscles are spared complete dependence on the mechanisms that deliver oxygen from air. This interplay between the role of the anaerobic and aerobic pathways in supplying ATP is important at workloads above 40 % of VO2max. Above this workload, the ATP turnover is faster than the rate of the creatine phosphate shuttle.

The level of creatine phosphate decreases linearly as exercise intensity increases. In addition, the level of effort corresponding to the onset of blood lactate accumulation has been shown to be closely related to performance capacity (Farrell et al., 1979; Sjödin & Jacobs, 1981). It is also documented that the absolute as well as the relative exercise intensity at which blood lactate starts to accumulate is higher for endurance-trained subjects than for sedentary subjects (MacDougall, 1977).

The decline in muscle strength and mass during ageing (MacDougall, 1977; Larson, Grimby & Karlson, 1979) has been linked to reduction in metabolic function. Dynamic exercise increases the aerobic metabolism of the exercising skeletal muscles in proportion to the mass of muscles and intensity of exertion involved. Skeletal muscle atrophy is often considered a hallmark of ageing, and this deficit has profound implications for the regeneration of ATP in the muscles. Oxidative capacity declines in some skeletal muscles with advancing age (Aniansson et al., 1983). Ageing is associated with alterations in body composition such that there is an increase in percentage of body fat and a concomitant decline in lean body mass. Thus, a significant loss in maximal force production takes place with ageing (Farrar, Martin & Ardies, 1981; Aniansson et al., 1986). These changes in muscle mass and strength may be due to alteration in the distribution of fibre types as a result of an interconversion between type I and type II muscle fibres or secondary to the preferential loss of a specific muscle fibre type (Stalberg et al., 1989). This is not a consistent finding, however, and some controversy in recent findings (Green, 1986; Lexell, Downham & Sjöstrom, 1986) suggest that when a loss of skeletal muscle mass occurs during ageing, it is not because of the preferential loss of a specific fibre type; both type I and type II skeletal muscle are equally affected. Electromyographic studies indicate the loss of fast-twitch neurons (Lexell et al., 1983), and fast-twitch neurons may be more susceptible to damage arising from local ischemia due to atherosclerotic lesions in the peripheral circulation (Campbell, McComas & Petito, 1973; Sjöstrom, Angquist & Rais, 1980). The selective loss of type II fibres would help to explain the reduced ability of the elderly to perform anaerobic tasks and would explain the discrepancy between muscle volume loss and the loss of strength, as well as the moderate loss of endurance ability in the face of a significant loss of strength.

Loss of muscle fibres and speed of movement may not be uniform throughout the body. It has been suggested that the muscles of the legs are affected to a greater degree by atrophy (Sjöstrom et al., 1982). In addition, blood flow in exercising muscle is lower in older (52 - 59 yrs.) men at every submaximal workload. Leg blood flow was 4.46 l . min^{-1} in maximal exercise for the older men, compared with 5.57 l . min^{-1} in the younger (25 - 30 yrs.) men at a lower, submaximal workload (Tomonag, 1977). This would reduce the ability of older subjects to increase VO2 uptake (in contrast to young individuals), since leg blood flow increases linearly during submaximal exercise with increasing workload and VO2. The effect of training on muscle blood flow during exercise has not been reported for old animals or humans.

For any individual, the specific metabolic requirements of a given exercise depend on a number of variables. One important variable is the mode of exercise, i.e., whether exercise is dynamic or static (and the active muscle mass). In prolonged submaximal effort, the duration of performance is markedly affected by the relation between exercise intensity and selection of metabolic fuel. At exercise intensities below the anaerobic threshold, plasma, free-fatty acids (FFA) and blood glucose are the primary oxidative substrate (Wahren et al., 1974). With increasing exercise intensity there is, however, a progressive increase in carbohydrate relative to lipid oxidation, and muscle glycogen dominates fuel for work (Ahlborg et al., 1974). In young subjects during moderate levels of energy metabolism, sufficient oxygen is available to the cells. Consequently, most of the substrates are oxidised within the mitochondria. In this case, lactic acid does not build up because its removal rate equals its rate of production. Since oxygen is essential for mitochondrial ATP production and since the main function of glycolysis is to supplement the production of ATP when oxidative processes do not meet the energetic demand, it seems that the elderly who have a diminished oxygen supply during submaximal exercise will elevate lactate concentration in blood and muscle (Saltin & Karlsson, 1971; Paffenbarger et al., 1993) to a higher level when compared to younger subjects while performing the same workload as percentage of VO2max.

Training effect on cardiopulmonary function and muscle metabolism

Performance of the heart as a pump has been a major element in testing the idea that exercise ameliorates the ageing process. Exercise training was associated with health benefits and specifically with decreased cardiovascular mortality in two large observational studies (Sandvik et al., 1993; Hull et al., 1994). Recently (Douglas & O'Toole, 1992), it was suggested that following training the mechanism most likely to be involved is a change in the cardiac autonomic balance, producing an increase, or a relative dominance, of the vagal component. It has been long known that exercise training reduces resting and submaximal heart rate. Several cardiac changes accompany the normal ageing process, including: the prolongation of excitation- contraction and relaxation, and an increase in afterload, increased vascular and myocardial stiffness, and decreased catecholamine sensitivity (Dehn & Bruce, 1972) .

Alterations in left ventricular structure and function are a well-described and accepted component of the response to physical conditioning. This is true if elderly or younger subjects are engaged in similar endurance training. Both age groups demonstrated cardiac changes previously documented to occur with exercise training, including lower heart rates, larger ventricular cavities, lower wall stresses, and higher passive/active phases ratio. Despite the occurrence of structural and functional changes in response to exercise in the older individuals hearts, the older hearts were significantly different in some respects from those of their younger counterparts, suggesting that some aspects of normal ageing were unaltered by exercise training.

The training effect on cardiopulmonary function during submaximal exercise of a fixed absolute work rate is similar for younger and older individuals. Although many studies have shown a decrease in functional capacity and VO2max among the ageing, it generally did not involve physically active older men.

A study (Heath et al., 1981) which compared physically active and sedentary men aged 40 to 72 years, suggested a significantly greater decrease in VO2max among those who were sedentary. Heath et al. (1981) has shown an almost twofold greater decline in VO2max per decade in sedentary subjects compared to active men (9 % vs. 5 %, respectively) after age 25. The degree of the VO2max improvement with training in the elderly, expressed in relative terms, appears to be comparable to that demonstrated by younger subjects. The increased VO2max in the active subjects may be due to an increase in mitocondrial respiratory capacity.

Variable	Rest	Sub-maximal Exercise	Maximal Exercise
Oxygen uptake	unchanged	unchanged	increases
Systolic blood pressure	decreases	decreases	decreases
Diastolic blood pressure	decreases	decreases	decreases
Stroke volume	decreases	increases	increases
Heart rate	decreases	decreases	unchanged
Cardiac output	unchanged	unchanged	increases
Contractility	unchanged	unchanged	unchanged /increase
Total peripheral resistance	unchanged	unchanged	decreases
Arteriovenous O2 difference	unchanged	unchanged	increases

Table 1: Endurance training-induced changes in cardiovascular and hemodynamic variables in elderly subjects.

Table 1 summarises some of the changes associated with age and training on cardiovascular and hemodynamic variables. Endurance exercise training in the elderly decreased resting and submaximal exercise heart rate, systolic and diastolic blood pressure, while stroke volume increased. Marked changes are notable in elderly subjects during maximal effort in which stroke volume, cardiac output, contractility, and oxygen uptake are increased, while total peripheral resistance, systolic and diastolic blood pressure decreased, thus lowering after-load which in turn facilitate left ventricular systolic and diastolic function.

Variable	Rest	Sub-maximal Exercise	Maximal Exercise
Maximal voluntary ventilation	unchanged	—	—
Maximal oxygen uptake	unchanged	unchanged	increases
Minute ventilation	unchanged	decreases	increases
Ventilation/ Oxygen uptake	unchanged	decreases	decreases
Ventilation/ Volume CO2	unchanged	unchanged	decreases
Lactic acid	unchanged	decreases	decreases

Table 2: Endurance training-induced changes in pulmonary function in elderly subjects.

Table 2 reveals that efficiency of breathing is improved in the elderly following an endurance training program. These changes include reduction in lactic acid levels and increased maximal ventilation. The most important adaptive response of skeletal muscle to endurance exercise is an augmentation of respiratory capacity with increases in the ability to oxidise pyruvate, fatty acids and ketones. As a result of increases in the levels of the enzymes of the malate-asparate shuttle, there is also an enhancement of the capability for mitochondrial oxidation of the reducing equivalents generated in the cytoplasm during glycolysis. The rise in muscle respiratory capacity results from an increase in muscle mitochondria and an alteration in mitochondrial composition, making skeletal muscle mitochondria more like heart mitochondria in their enzyme pattern (Saltin & Rowell, 1980).

When previously sedentary individuals are re-tested at the same absolute submaximal work rate after adapting to endurance exercise, their endurance is found to be markedly increased (Sagiv et al., 1989). However, metabolic factors do not appear to determine the magnitude of VO2max.

The changes in muscle oxidative potential may play a major role in the capacity of elderly to perform submaximal work. As an example, in physically conditioned young subjects, submaximal work performance increased by 300 % while VO2max increased 19 % (Holloszy & Booth, 1976).

In conclusion, these data indicate that the skeletal muscle, cardiovascular system and pulmonary function of older persons retain a high degree of trainability, with much of the improvement occurring peripherally, just as in younger individuals.

References
(* denotes references which would be of particular interest to non-specialists)

Ahlborg, G., Felig, P., Hagenfeldt, L., Hendler, R., Wahren, R. (1974). Substrate turnover during prolonged exercise in men splanchnic and leg metabolism of glucose, free fatty acids and amino acids. *Journal of Clinical Investigation,* 53: 1080-1090.

Aniansson, A., Hedberg, M., Henning, G.B., Grimby, G. (1986). Muscle morphology, enzymatic activity, and muscle strength in elderly men: A follow-up study. *Muscle Nerve,* 9: 585-591.

Aniansson, A., Sperling, L., Rundgren, A., Lehnberg, E. (1983). Muscle function in 75-year-old men and women. *Scandinavian Journal of Rehabilitative Medicine Supplement,* 9: 92-102.

Bertel, O., Buhler, F.R., Klowski, W., Lutold, B.E. (1980). Decreased beta-adrenoreceptor responsiveness as related to age, blood pressure, and plasma catecholamines in patients with essential hypertension. *Hypertension,* 2: 130-138.

Black, L.E. & Hyatt, R.E. (1969). Maximal respiratory pressures: Normal values and relationship to age and sex. *American Review of Respiratory Disorders,* 99: 696-702.

Booth, F.W., Weeden, S.H., Tseng, B.S. (1994). Effect of ageing on human skeletal muscle and motor function. *Medicine and Science in Sports and Exercise,* 26: 556-560.

Campbell, M.J., McComas, A.J., Petito, F. (1973). Physiological changes in ageing muscles. *Journal of Neurology, Neurosurgery and Psychiatry,* 36: 174-182.

Capasso, J.M., Puntillo, E., Olivetti, G., Anversa, P. (1989). Difference in load dependence of relaxation between the left and right ventricular myocardium as a function of age in rats. *Circulation Research,* 65: 1499-1507.

Conway, J., Wheeler, R., Sannerstedt, R. (1971). Sympathetic nervous activity during exercise in relation to age. *Cardiovascular Research,* 5:577-581.

Dehn, M.M. & Bruce, R.A. (1972). Longitudinal variations in maximal oxygen uptake with age and activity. *Journal of Applied Physiology,* 33: 805-807.

Dempsey, J. (1987). Exercise-induced imperfections in pulmonary gas exchange. *Canadian Journal of Applied Sport Science,* 12: 665-705.

Douglas, P.S. & O'Toole, M. (1992). Ageing and physical activity determine cardiac structure and function in the older athlete. *Journal of Applied Physiology,* 72: 1969-1973.

Downes, R.T., Nomeir, A.M., Smith, M.K., Stewart, P.K., Little, C.M. (1989). Mechanism of altered pattern of left ventricular filling with ageing in subjects without cardiac disease. *American Journal of Cardiology,* 64: 523-27.

Ehsani, A.A., Ogana, T., Miller, T.R., Spina, R.J., Jilka, S.M. (1991). Exercise training improves left ventricular systolic function in older men. *Circulation,* 8: 96-103.

Farrar, R.P., Martin, T.P., Ardies, C.M. (1981). The interaction of ageing and endurance exercise upon the mitochondrial function of skeletal muscle. *Journal of Gerontology,* 36: 642-647.

Farrell, P.A., Wilmore, J.H., Coyle, E.F., Billing, J.E., Costill, D.L. (1979). Plasma lactate accumulation and distance running performance. *Medicine and Science in Sports,* 11: 338-344.

Fleg, J. & Lakatta, E.G. (1988). Role of muscle role. In the age-associated reduction in VO2max.. *Journal of Applied Physiology,* 65: 1147-1151.

Gardin, J.M., Rohan, M.K., Davidsen, D.M., et al. (1987). Doppler transmitral flow velocity parameters: Relationship between age, body surface area, blood pressure and gender in normal subjects. *American Journal of Noninvasive Cardiology*, 1: 3-10.

Green, H.J. (1986). Characteristics of ageing human muscle. Sutton, J.R., Brook, R.M. (eds.). *Sports Medicine for the Mature Athlete*. Indianapolis, In: Benchmark Press. pp. 12-26.

Hagberg, J.M., Graves, J.E., Limalkcher, M., et al. (1989). Cardiovascular responses of 70 to 79-yr-old men and women to exercise training. *Journal of Applied Physiology*, 66: 2589-2594.

Heath, G.W., Hagberg, J.M., Ehsani, A.A. et al. (1981). A physiological comparison of young and older endurance athletes. *Journal of Applied Physiology*, 51: 634-640.

Hoeldtke, R.D. & Cilms, K.M. (1985). Effects of ageing on catecholamine metabolism. *Journal of Clinical Endocrinology Metabolism*, 60: 479-484.

Holloszy, J.O. & Booth, F.W. (1976). Biochemical adaptations to endurance training in muscle. *Annual Review of Physiology*, 38: 273-291.

Hull, S.S., Vanoli, E., Adamson, P.B., Verrier, R.L., Foreman, R.D., Schwartz, P.J. (1994). Exercise training confers anticipatory protection from sudden death during acute myocardial ischemia. *Circulation*, 89: 548-552.

Islam, M.S. (1980). Mechanism of controlling residual volume and emptying rate of the lung in young and elderly healthy subjects. *Respiration*, 40: 1-8.

Johnson, B.D. & Dempsey, J.A. (1991). Demand vs capacity in the ageing pulmonary system. In: *Exercise and Sport Sciences Reviews*. Holloszy, J.O. (Ed.) Baltimore, Williams & Wilkins. pp. 171-210.

Johnson, B.D., Reddan, W.G., Pegelow, D.F., Seow, K.C., Dempsey, J.A. (1991a). Flow limitation and regulation of functional residual capacity during exercise in a physically active ageing population. *American Review of Respiratory Disorders*, 143: 960-967.

Johnson, B.D., Reddan, W.G., Seow, K.C., Dempsey, J.A. (1991b). Mechanical constraints on exercise hyperpnea in a fit ageing population. *American Review of Respriatory Disorders,* 143: 968-977.

Kallinen, M., Suominen, H., Vuolteenaho, O., Alen, M. (1998). Effort tolerance in elderly women with different physical activity backgrounds. *Medicine and Science in Sports and Exercise,* 30: 170-176.

Krumpe, P.E., Knudson, R.J., Parsons, G., Reiser, K. (1985). The ageing respiratory system. *Clinical Gerontology Medicine,* 1: 143-175.

Kuo, L.C., Quinones, M.A., Rokey, R., Sartori, M., Abinader, E.G., Zoghb,i W.A. (1987). Quantification of aerial contribution to left ventricular filling by pulsed Doppler echocardiography and the effect of age in normal and diseased hearts. *American Journal of Cardiology,* 59: 1147-78.

Lakatta, E.G. (1993). Deficient neuroendocrine regulation of the cardiovascular system with advancing age in healthy humans. *Circulation,* 87: 631-636.

Larson, K., Grimby, G., Karlsson, J. (1979). Muscle strength and speed of movement in relation to age and muscle morphology. *Journal of Applied Physiology,* 46: 451-456.

Levitzky, M.G. (1984). Effects of ageing on the respiratory system. *The physiologist,* 27: 102-106.

Lexell, J., Downham, D.Y., Sjöstrom, M. (1986). Distribution of different fiber types in human skeletal muscle: Fiber type arrangement in m. vastus lateralis from three groups of healthy men between 15 and 83 years. *Journal of Neurological Sciences,* 72: 211-222.

Lexell, J., Hendriksson-Larsen, K., Winblad, B., Sjöstrom, M. (1983). Distribution of different fiber types in human skeletal muscles: Effects of ageing studied in whole muscle cross section. *Muscle Nerve,* 6: 588-595.

MacDougall, J.H. (1977). The anaerobic threshold: Its significance for the endurance athlete. *Canadian Journal of Applied Sport Sciences*, 2: 137-140.

Mauderly, J.L. & Hahn, F.F. (1982). The effects of age on lung function and structure of adult animals. Advances in Veterinarian. Science Comparative Medicine, 26: 35-77.

*Paffenbarger, R.S., Hyde, R.T., Wing, A.L., Lee, J., Jung, D.L., Kampert, J.B. (1993). The association of changes in physical activity level and other lifestyle characteristics with mortality among men. *New England Journal of Medicine*, 328: 538-545.

Pollock, M.L., Foster, C., Knapp, D., Rod, J.L., Schmidt, D.H. (1987). Effect of age and training in aerobic capacity and body composition of master athletes. *Journal of Applied Physiology,* 62: 725-731.

Rodeheffer, R.G., Gerstenblith, G., Becker, L.C., Fleg, J.L., Weisfelt, M.L., Lakatta, E.G. (1984). Exercise cardiac output is maintained with advancing age in healthy human subjects: Cardiac dilatation and increases stroke volume compensate for a diminished heart rate. *Circulation*, 69: 203-213.

*Rodgers, M.A., Wagberg, J.M., Martin III, W.H., Ehsani, A.A., Holloszy, J.O. (1990). Decline in VO2max with ageing in master athletes and sedentary men. *Journal of Applied Physiology,* 68: 2195-2199.

Sagiv, M., Goldhammer, E., Ben-Sira, D. (1992). Effect of increased after-load on left ventricular filling properties in healthy elderly and young subjects. *Medicine Exercise Nutrition and Health*, 1: 48-53.

*Sagiv, M., Fisher, N., Yaniv, A., Ruddy, J. (1989). Effect of running versus isometric training programs on healthy elderly at rest. *Gerontology*, 35: 72-77.

Sagiv, M., Goldhammer, E., Abinader, E.G., Rudoy, J. (1986). Ageing and the effect of increased after-load on left ventricular contractile state. *Medicine and Science in Sports and Exercise,* 20: 281-284.

Saltin, B. & Karlsson, J. (1971). Muscle glycogen utilization during work of different intensities. In Pernow, B., Saltin, B. (eds.). *Advances in experimental medicine and biology*. VI. 11. Muscle metabolism during exercise. New York. Plenum Press. 289-299.

*Saltin, B. & Rowell, L.B. (1980). Functional adaptations to physical activity and inactivity. *Federation Proceedings.*, 39: 1506-1513.

Sandvik, L., Erikssen, J., Thaulow, E., Erikssen, O., Mundal, R., Rodahl, K. (1993). Physical Fitness as a predictor of mortality among healthy, middle-aged Norwegian men. *New England Journal of Medicine,* 328: 574-575.

*Shephard, R.J. (1989). The ageing of cardiovascular function. In: *Physical Activity and Ageing*. Spirduso, W.W., Eckert, H.M. (Eds.). Champaign, IL: Human Kinetics. pp. 175-185.

*Shephard, R.J. (1987). *Physical Activity and Ageing* (2nd ed.). London: Croom Helm.

Sjödin, B. & Jacobs, I. (1981). Onset of blood lactate accumulation and marathon running performance. *International Journal of Sports Medicine*, 2: 23-26.

Sjöstrom, M., Neglen, P., Friden, J., Eklof, B. (1982). Human skeletal muscle metabolism and morphology after temporary incomplete ischemia. *European Journal of Clinical Investigation*, 12: 69-79.

Sjöstrom, M., Angquist, K.A., Rais, O. (1980). Intermittent claudication and muscle fiber fine structure: Correlation between clinical and morphological data. *Ultrastructure Pathology*, 1: 309-326.

Stalberg, R., Borges, O., Ericcson, M., Essen-Gustavsson, B., Fawcett, P., Nordesjo, L., Nordgren Uhlin, R. (1989). The quadriceps femoris muscle in 20-70-year old subjects: Relationship between knee extension torque electrophysiological parameters, and muscle fiber characteristics. *Muscle Nerve*, 12: 382-389.

Stoddard, M.F., Pearson, A.L., Kern, M.J., Atcleeiff, J., Mrosek, D.G., Labovitz, A.J. (1989). Influence of alteration in preload on the pattern of left ventricular diastolic filling as assessed by Doppler echocardiography in humans. *Circulation*, 79: 1226-36.

Tate, C.A., Hyek, M.F., Taffet, G.E. (1994). Mechanisms for the responses of cardiac muscle to physical activity in old age. *Medicine and Science in Sports and Exercise*, 26: 561-567.

Tate, C.A., Taffet, G.E., Hudson, E.D., Blaylock, S.L., McBride, R.P., Michael, L.H. (1990). Enhanced calcium uptake of cardiac sarcoplasmic reticulum in exercise-trained rats. *American Journal of Physiology*, 258: H431-435.

Tomonag, M. (1977). Histochemical and ultrastructual changes in senile human skeletal muscle. *Journal of the American Geriatric Society*, 25: 125-131.

Wahren, J., Saltin, B., Jorfeldt, L., Pernow, B. (1974). Influence of age on the local circulatory adaptation to leg exercise. *Scandinavian Journal of Clinical and Laboratory Investigation*, 33: 79-86.

Weisfeldt, M.L., Gerstenblith, G. (1986). Cardiovascular ageing and adaptation to disease. In: *The Heart*, 6th ed. Hust, J.W. (Ed.) New York: McGraw-Hill Book Co. pp. 1403-1411.

Physical Activity and Ageing: A Perspective in Developing Countries

Sandra Mahecha Matsudo and Victor Keihan Rodrigues Matsudo

Ageing in Latin America: an Overview

Ageing of populations is a global phenomenon affecting rich and developing countries alike. Data surveyed by the Pan-American Health Organization (PAHO, 1997) show a new Latin American scenario where the countries with the largest ratio of individuals older than 60 are Uruguay (17.3 %), Argentina, and Puerto Rico (13.8 %). From 1997 to 2025, in Latin America the countries expected to experience the most striking growth rates in their 60-year-plus populations are the following: French Guyana (289 %), Nicaragua (229 %), Colombia (221 %), Venezuela (216 %), and Costa Rica (207 %). Brazil ranks sixteenth among these nations, and is likely to rise by 163 %. From 1950 to 2025, the number of elderly in Brazil must eventually increase by as much as fifteen times, whereas the population at large will only grow by five times. This will place Brazil in sixth position world-wide in terms of number of elders, who will account for 32 million people in 2025. Brazil's 1997 figures for life expectancy at birth were 57 years for males and 66 years for females. Life expectancy for the average Brazilian is projected at 80 years for both women and men within the period 2000 to 2025.

As part of a drive to attend to these new realities, both governmental and non-governmental organisations in Brazil have been making efforts to

Correspondence to: Dr. Sandra Matsudo, Physical Fitness Research Center of São Caetano do Sul – CELAFISCS, The Agita São Paulo Program, Sao Caetano do Sul, Av. Goiás, 1400, 09520 São Paulo, Brazil promote healthy ageing. Among these actions is the implementation of policies to specifically meet the needs of these populations in order to maintain and/or rehabilitate their functional abilities. Also included are campaigns run by the Federal Health Department recently such as *Viver Mais e Melhor ("Live Healthier and Longer")*. The programme provided this community with a guide suggesting the best ways to live its life better and with improved quality, adding recommendations on basic health care maintenance, nutrition, exercise, and social and citizenship-related activities.

In the Brazilian states, there are a number of Departments developing specific programmes to care for those older than 60. The state administration has set as a top priority the integration of these programmes or projects under development to accomplish an articulated care programme for elders. As a result, the different state departments responsible for health, culture, social assistance and development, sport and tourism, housing, transportation, environment, agriculture, justice, labour, and education, began looking at this issue from a intersectoral approach to give elders integral, appropriate care.

From the point of view of active ageing, there are specific programmes being developed by a number of these Departments for the elderly population. The Social Assistance and Development Department has been implementing home care programmes including both open and residential activities to promote relationships and conviviality and respect for individuality, autonomy and independence, to strengthen family links and prevent institutionalisation. The Culture Department has conducted programmes through cultural workshops dealing with art and culture from such varied standpoints as learning foreign languages, music, painting, dancing, drawing, composition, role playing, tai chi, singing, and so on. Also handling these themes, the Sport and Tourism Department has an "Elderly People's Club" featuring cultural, sporting, tourism and recreation activities. And such non-governmental organisations as SESI (Industry's Social Service) and SESC (Commerce's Social Service) have also been organising health and recreation-oriented services for Brazilian elders.

Physical Activity and Ageing

The diagnostic assessment process in the Agita São Paulo Program conducted in Greater São Paulo and other cities in the state has identified knowledge levels, barriers and facilitation means in connection with exercise. In a sample of the state population, we surveyed the reasons for elders allegedly refraining from carrying out exercise on a regular basis. The data found suggest that the most frequent barriers preventing physical activity, according to gender, in São Paulo State's small towns are as follows:

Females	Males
1. No equipment	1. No equipment
2. Need for rest	2. No proper location
3. No proper location	3. Inability
4. Weather conditions	4. Weather conditions
5. Inability	5. Need for rest

For the capital and cities in Greater São Paulo with more than 500,000 inhabitants, the most frequent barriers were found to be the following:

1. No equipment
2. No time available
3. Lack of knowledge
4. Fear of being physically harmed
5. Need for rest

The survey clearly shows that barriers vary according to gender and city size. A common element in these barriers, however, is that they are far from involving reasons of poor health or unwillingness. Rather, they could be easily resolved by dissemination of new messages encouraging physical activity. These messages indicate that one does not need special equipment, locations, abilities, or knowledge to be active on a regular basis. Considering the environmental factors that help elders get involved in regular physical activity, those older than 50 are recommended or advised to exercise by the sources in next table in the following order of priority:

Females	Males
1. Physician (38.3 %)	1. Physician (50.3 %)
2. Friends (33.3 %)	2. Friends (25.8 %)
3. Family (10.4 %)	3. Company (7.0 %)
4. Company (10.4 %)	4. Agita São Paulo Program (7.0 %)
5. Co-workers (4.2 %)	5. Family (6.3 %)
6. Agita São Paulo Program (3.3 %)	6. Co-workers (3.5 %)

The level of knowledge about the new physical activity standards for health promotion has been found to differ based on the surveyed gender and location. The new physical activity paradigm for health promotion advocates that individuals should exercise moderately at least 30 minutes a day on most days of the week or every day, if they can, either successively or on an accumulative basis. This diagnosis is based upon a questionnaire that was applied in several São Paulo State cities. In smaller towns only 32 % of females and 35 % of males were determined to reach the new physical activity knowledge standard. Nevertheless, nearly 36 % of women and 31 % of men said they thought that physical activity should be conducted three to four times a week, with sessions longer than 30 minutes. In Greater São Paulo and other cities in the state, the results proved to be relatively better – around 40 % of females and 51 % of males responded according to the new paradigm.

Interestingly, however, there was a relationship encountered between knowledge and the physical activity levels of elderly people. In cities with more inhabitants, less than 23 % of those familiar with the new paradigm carried out exercises according to the new recommendations. Of these, 25 % (males) and 32 % (females) were irregularly active, and 48 % of women and 53 % of men were sedentary. In smaller towns the findings are more serious, as only 14 % of individuals familiar with the new paradigm perform physical activity to these recommendations. Among women, 34 % were irregularly active and 41 % sedentary. Of men, 25.2 % were irregularly active and nearly 40 % sedentary. The evidence collected strongly indicates that a proper level of knowledge does not necessarily result in regular involvement on the basis of the new physical activity paradigms. This goes to show that promotion of physical activity should bring with it an emphasis not only on increasing the level of knowledge, but also developing strategies to overcome the barriers hindering active lifestyles.

Physical Fitness, Training and Ageing

Since 1974, the Physical Fitness Research Center from São Caetano do Sul (CELAFISCS) has been developing various investigations to assess how physical activity, physical fitness, training and ageing relate to one another. For the last five years our projects have aimed at two major areas: 1) To study the effects of training programmes for muscle strength, gymnastics programmes using lifting weights and tai chi on the physical fitness of sedentary women; and 2) To study how physical fitness and functional abilities progress in active elderly women.

1. Training and Ageing. The results of different types of muscle strength training programmes using devices and free lifting weights, fabricated from common materials, with groups consisting of the community's sedentary women, proved beneficial. The most important effects were the improvement of some physical activity neuromotor variables (the muscle strength of both upper and lower limbs), especially such physical functioning as walking speed, balance and stair climbing speed. The tai chi programmes, held once a week, yielded results that enable us to find significantly improved balance, walking speed and trunk flexibility. While this improvement is important from a statistical standpoint, the data are only relevant with a few of the variables studied, as they mean not only that key variables of the everyday life's activities have improved but especially that physical activity's anthropometric and neuromotor variables have been maintained.

2. Progress of Physical Fitness and Ageing. In 1996, CELAFISCS started the Longitudinal Physical Fitness and Ageing Project in São Caetano do Sul - the only one in developing countries. Every six months physically active, independent, elderly women in the community are evaluated for physical fitness (anthropometric and neuromotor variables), physical functioning, nutritional ingestion profile, physical activity levels, and psychological variables (body image, mood, and depression). The first results of the evaluations conducted in the year following the baseline show that most variables tended to be maintained, regardless of the age group (50-59, 60-69, or 70-79 years). For the walking speed and standing up speed from the chair, most age groups experienced considerable improvement during the one-year period. On the other

hand, both flexibility and balance diminished significantly on the 70-plus group. These findings suggest how different the effect of the ageing process is on the physical fitness and physical function variables of active elderly women, depending upon their age.

Promotion of Physical Activity in the Elderly Population –
The Agita São Paulo Program Experience

The state of São Paulo has around 34 million inhabitants, spread over 645 municipalities. As many as 17 million people live in the capital, São Paulo City, and in Greater São Paulo alone. These figures suggest how strongly noncommunicable chronic diseases such as cardiovascular problems, cancer, diabetes, chronic obstructive pulmonary diseases and mental disorders can impact on public health. These conditions account for 47.3 % of deaths in the state, 38.4 % of which were before 60 years of age. They are the chief causes for adult disability and account for over 50 % of retirement cases due to declining physical functioning. In 70 % of the cases, nevertheless, the key factors are environmental or behavioural in nature and thus could be controlled by comparatively straightforward actions.

Inferences can be drawn that sedentary habits are the prevalent risk factors among the population, regardless of gender. Quite obviously, this underscores the importance of having active ways of life that in turn somehow will control and reduce the other risk factors. The positive relationship of physical activity and reduced mortality is evidenced in epidemiological and experimental investigations. Some of its benefits are decreased risks of cardiovascular diseases, improved profile of plasmatic lipids, sustained bone density, reduced pain in the hips, and a positive outlook of more control over chronic pulmonary diseases. Also, positive effects have been reported on the primary or complementary treatment of arteriosclerosis, poor peripheral venous tone, osteoporosis, and arthritis, as well as psychological benefits produced both in the short term, such as decreased anxiety and stress, and in the long term such as shifted moderate depression, mood, self-esteem, self-image, socialisation, and positive attitudes. And since physical activity by the elderly helps reduce the risk of falls and ameliorates balance and muscle strength, it also helps people maintain physical functioning and thus minimises the effects of physical decline, insomnia, excessive consumption of medicines, and social isolation. Against this background, the São Paulo State Health Department requested the Physical Fitness Research Center from São Caetano do Sul (CELAFISCS) to develop a programme to promote health via physical activity. This program has been prepared over two years, with support from the Pan American Health Organization, US Centers for Disease Control (CDC), English Health Education Authority, and the Institute for Aerobic Research in Dallas, Texas. This programme is backed by a group of scientific advisers and partner institutions (Figure 1). It is formed by professionals having broad experience in sports sciences from both our research centre and the most important Brazilian universities. Also participating are 144 governmental and non-governmental organisations which play a part in the Executive Board. This is the forum where both community and individual actions are discussed and the general event calendar is set up. Based on this framework, the Agita São Paulo Program has three main targets for its strategic actions: Students (both children and adolescents), workers (both blue- and white-collar), and elders.

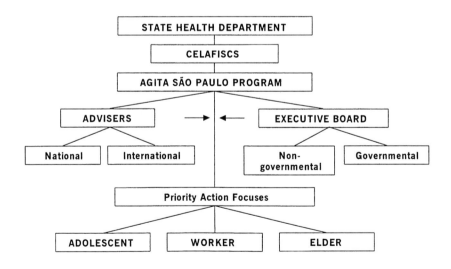

Figure 1. Function Organization of the Agita São Paulo Program

Objectives of the Agita São Paulo Program

At an early stage, the major objective of the program is to encourage awareness; in the long term, actions will be directed to effectively striving to change the behaviour of the São Paulo state population. This can be summarised as follows:

1. Increase the population's knowledge levels about the benefits of an active lifestyle.
2. Increase the population's physical activity levels.

As an aid for hitting these targets an Action Model (Figure 2) has been designed for the Program to describe and help understand how actions should be taken towards the community and the diagnostic evaluation process and how successful the Program is.

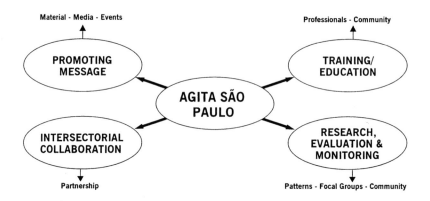

Figure 2. Strategic Planning Model For Evaluation - Agita São Paulo Conceptual Model

As can be seen from this Model, the main activities of the Program focus on eight key areas:

1. Dissemination of the Message via Media
2. Professional/Training Education Lectures
3. Direct Community Education
4. Community Education through trained Professionals
5. Coalition Building/Intersectoral Collaboration

6. Resource/Material Production
7. Community Events
8. Research, Evaluation, Monitoring

The specific activities are included in Chart 1 below:

---

1. Dissemination of the Message via Media
For the most part, unpaid message promotion in:
- Newspapers
- TV/radio Interviews
- Posters
- Folders

2 Professional/Training Education Lectures
Especially meant for health professionals or those in direct connection with the community:
- Physicians, nurses
- Physical education professionals
- Teachers
- Others

3. Direct Community Education to Community
This activity will be performed by the Program's professionals and will be targeted at:
- Elders
- Adolescents, students
- Adults
- Workers

4. Community Education Delivered by Trained Professionals
This will be accomplished using
- Lectures
- Promotional material

5. Coalition Building/Intersectoral Collaboration
This has been the most valuable and far-reaching strategy to promote the Program's message and actions. Partnership is established with different governmental and non-governmental organisations that promote all the activities mentioned herein with no need for additional funding. Among these partnerships aimed at promoting the message within the group of elders are the elderly centres, elderly club associations, state education, sporting, culture, social assistance, health, industry/commerce social service departments, the Rotary, the Lions, medical associations, public, private and elderly universities, and municipalities.

6. Resource/Material Production
Development of high-quality, effective material:
- Posters
- Flyers
- Folders
- Mousepads, pencils, T-shirts

- Manual, transparencies
- Courses/training

This material is also prepared on the basis of the Program's focuses and the message that will be disseminated. There are also specific folders and posters intended for the people older than 60 years according to their characteristics and requirements.

7. **Community Events**
Primarily:
- Agita initiated events
- Agita taking part in events initiated by others

The Program's super-events include one annual event that takes place at the same time as the National or International Day of Older Persons. The organisation starts at least six months ahead with the entities involved in elderly work as partners. This event often comprises a walk of no more than 11/2 miles around strategic locations in town. When the group gathers together following the walk, a recreational/cultural activity is carried out. Material containing information on the Program is given away and the message is transmitted to everyone at all times, encouraging active ways of life. The significance of inter-generational relations is highlighted and elders are strongly prompted to have as much contact with their relatives and friends as they can.

8. **Research, Evaluation, Monitoring**
From the start, subjects undergo a comprehensive diagnostic evaluation for physical activity levels, knowledge levels about physical activity and health, and motivation and barriers to physical activity. This diagnosis has been used especially with elderly centres, homes, elderly care centres, and this age group in general.

Chart 1: Key activities of the Agita São Paulo Program

Specific Activities with Elders

Since 1996, the Agita São Paulo Program has been developing specific activities with elderly people, as shown in Chart 2.

1. Increase the population's knowledge about the health benefits from active lifestyle
2. Encourage regular exercise for elders
3. Diagnostically determine knowledge levels about physical activity and existing elderly physical activity levels
4. Once a year participate and help organise a walk to celebrate the International Day of Older Persons. In 1999, the International Year of Older Persons, the Program took part in the committee in charge of setting up in São Paulo the WHO/OMS-supported event the Global Embrace on October 2. In São Paulo State we gathered as partners to get the municipality's capabilities in place for this world event.
5. Prepare a manual to promote the Program's activities with the state's elderly population. This would be designed to communicate to the professionals involved in this work of physical activity benefits for elders and put together objectives and strategies to implement physical activity programmes among independent and dependent as well as institutionalised and non-institutionalised individuals.

6. Promote the use of city areas to perform elderly-oriented activities.
7. Motivate elders to take a new active approach in three contexts: in the home, in the workplace, and in free hours.
8. Train human resources to design regular physical activity programmes reflecting the elderly population's realities.

Chart 2. Agita São Paulo Program's Special Activities for Elders

The Program's Message

The latest scientific evidence shows that there is a new health promotion paradigm based on physical exercise. The new paradigms recommend active lifestyles as a means to enhance health. Such international entities as the World Health Organization (WHO/OMS); International Council of Sports Science and Physical Education (ICSSPE); US Center for Control and Prevention of Diseases (CDC); American College for Sports Medicine (ACSM); and International Sports Medicine Federation (FIMS) advocate conducting of moderate physical activities 30 minutes a day on most days of the week or every day consecutively, or on an accumulation basis. Focuses of these activities are the home, workplace and free time. This means elders should be encouraged to carry out daily tasks such as climbing up and down stairs, walking dogs, gardening, washing cars, strolling, dancing, cycling, and swimming. Chart 3 contains a number of Agita recommendations based on these new concepts.

• Use the stairs rather than the elevator
• Park your car further from your destination
• Step out of your train, bus or subway train one or two stations from your destination
• Instead of driving, walk to bank, supermarket, mall, and so on
• Take care of your house and garden yourself
• If you have a car, wash it yourself
• Go out dancing, or dance in your home, even if by yourself
• Get on your feet and shift to another TV channel, instead of using the remote control
• While you're watching TV, take the opportunity of stretching and weight lifting exercises
• Go shopping yourself
• While in a line in the bank or the post office, strengthen your abdomen and leg muscles
• Try to carry out some activities with your friends, relatives, or meeting centres, so you get more pleasure being active
• Remember that swimming, aquatics, chair exercise, yoga, tai chi, and other activities to strengthen your muscles are all beneficial and carry with them nearly no risks
• For those who can't, or find it hard to move, try stimulating activities such as stretching and strengthening of the arms and chest and abdominal muscles

Chart 3. Agita São Paulo Program Recommendations to Promote Active Elderly Lifestyle

Program Recommendations for Elders to Overcome Major Barriers to a More Active Lifestyle

A few suggestions can be given to break down the main physical activity barriers. They are:

Lack of Time
- You will spend only *30 minutes* a day, which can be cumulative. Just take the best from your hours and reduce more sedentary activities. Remember that you can exercise for successive time (all at once), or on an accumulative basis (for instance, 15 minutes plus 15 minutes, or ten minutes three times).

No Equipment, Inability, or Lack of Knowledge
- No piece of equipment, ability, or knowledge is specifically required for you to get more active. All you have to do is walk, dance, stroll around with your relatives or friends, walk your dog, garden, climb the stairs, and wash your car or bicycle.

There are a few things to keep in mind:
- You don't need to be in shape to begin getting active
- You don't need to leave your house to be active
- You don't need to have too much time to spare; the exercise activities can be performed on an accumulation basis during your everyday activities.

Conclusions and Prospects

While there are considerable socio-economic differences between the industrialised nations and the so-called developing countries, population ageing is a common phenomenon, arguably having a stronger impact on Latin America. Obviously, ageing is not the only problem facing our societies. Sedentary habits are, and will continue to be, the worst enemy of health as they are present in at least 50 % of the elderly population. The existing barriers clearly show that lacking appropriate knowledge about how to be physically active later in life can be the major reason for sedentary attitudes. This evidence is even more obvious when most of the elders say they cannot get involved in exercise more frequently because they have no equipment or they do not have enough physical ability to do so.

A portion of the population *is* aware of the new physical activity paradigm. And yet this is not reflected in the activities they perform in practice. Doctors and friends play a key role in encouraging and trying to make elders aware of this necessity. This means that these key groups should be taken into account when the physical activity programs intended for this age group are designed and developed.

Based on data from the Longitudinal Physical Fitness and Ageing Project that is now in progress, and from specific protocols that have been performed (muscle strength training and tai chi), regular physical activity is critical to maintain physical fitness and physical functioning for ageing individuals.

Experience with physical activity promotion programs such as "Agita São Paulo" or "Muevete Bogotá" has shown Latin America that health can be promoted using straightforward strategies, and it makes no difference if one begins being physically active daily when he or she moves into the elderly age range.

Acknowledgements

To Agita São Paulo Staff: Erinaldo Andrade, Timóteo Araújo, Douglas Andrade, Luis Oliveira, Aylton Figueira. Special gratitude to John Andrews for the English corrections.

References

American College Of Sports Medicine (1998). Position stand on exercise and physical activity for older adults. *Medicine and Science in Sport and Exercise*, 30, 992-1008.

Andrade, E., Matsudo, S., Matsudo, V., Araújo, T., Andrade, D., Oliveira, L., Figueira, A. (2000). Barriers and motivational factors for physical activity adherence in elderly people in developing country [abstract]. *Medicine and Science in Sport and Exercise*, 32, 141. [Presented at 47th American College of Sports Medicine Annual Meeting; 2000 May 31-Jun 3; Indianapolis (Indiana)].

Andrade, E., Matsudo, S., Matsudo, V., Araújo, T., Andrade, D., Figueira, Jr. A., Oliveira, L. (1999) Nível de atividade física de adultos acima de 50 anos de idade do estado de São Paulo. In: *Anais XXII Simpósio Internacional de Ciências do Esporte* (pp.125); 1999 Oct. 7-10. São Paulo, Brasil: Celafiscs.

Governo Do Estado De São Paulo-Secretaria de Estado da Saúde. (1998). *Programa Agita São Paulo*. São Paulo.

Matsudo, S., Andrade, E., Matsudo, V., Araújo, T., Barros, T. (2000). Evolution of neuromotor performance in active elderly women in one-year period as related to choronological age [abstract]. *Medicine and Science in Sport and Exercise*, 32, 219. [Presented at 47th American College of Sports Medicine Annual Meeting; 2000 May 31-Jun 3; Indianapolis (Indiana)].

Matsudo, S., Araújo, T., Andrade, E., Andrade, D., Matsudo, V., Barros, T. (1999). Evolution of neuromotor performance in active elderly women after 8-month period [abstract]. *Revista Antioqueña de Medicina Deportiva*, 2, 124.

Matsudo, S., Andrade, E., Matsudo, V., Andrade, D., Araújo, T., Figueira, Jr. A., Oliveira, L. (1999). Padrão de conhecimento do novo paradigma da atividade física de acordo com o nível de atividade física em idosos não sedentários do estado de São Paulo. In: *Anais XXII Simpósio Internacional de Ciências do Esporte* (pp. 125); Oct. 7-10. São Paulo, Brasil: Celafiscs.

Matsudo, S., Andrade, E., Matsudo, V., Araújo, T., Andrade, D., Figueira, A., Oliveira, L. (1999). Nível de atividade física em relação ao grau de conhecimento do novo paradigma da atividade física em indivíduos maiores de 50 anos. In: *Anais II Congresso Brasileiro de Atividade Física e Saúde* (pp. 143); Nov 24-26. Florianópolis, Brasil: NuPAF.

Matsudo, S., Andrade, E., Matsudo, V., Araújo, T., Andrade, D., Figueira, A., Oliveira, L. (1999). Nível de atividade física em relação ao grau de conhecimento do novo paradigma da atividade física em indivíduos maiores de 50 anos. In: *Anais II Congresso Brasileiro de Atividade Física e Saúde* (pp. 153); Nov 24-26. Florianópolis, Brasil: NuPAF.

Matsudo, S., Andrade, E., Araujo, T., Matsudo, V., Barros, T. (1998). Anthropometric and motor performance characteristics as related to age in active elderly women [abstract]. *Medicine and Science in Sport and Exercise,* 30 (5 Supl) 335. [Presented at 45th American College of Sports Medicine Annual Meeting; 1998 Jun 3-6; Orlando (Florida)].

Oliveira, R., Matsudo, S., Andrade, D., Matsudo, V. (1999). Effect of Tai-Chi-Chuan on physical fitness of elderly women [abstract]. *Medicine and Science in Sport and Exercise*, 31,385. [Presented at 46th American College of Sports Medicine Annual Meeting; 1999 Jun 2-5; Seattle (Washington)].

Organizacion Panamericana De La Salud. Instituto Nacional de Envejecimiento. *Envejecimiento en las Américas: proyecciones para el siglo XXI.* EUA; 1998.

Pate, R., Pratt, M., Blair, S., Haskell, W., Macera, C., Bouchard, C., Buchner, D., Ettinger, W., Heath, G., King, A., Kriska, A., Leon, A., Marcus, B., Morris, J., Paffenbarger, R., Patrick, K., Pollock, M., Rippe, J., Sallis, J., Wilmore, J. (1995). Physical activity and public health: A recommendation from the Center for Disease Control and Prevention and the American College of Sports Medicine. *Journal of the American Medical Association,* 273, 402-407.

Raso, V., Andrade, E., Matsudo, S., Matsudo, V. (1997). Exercício com pesos para mulheres idosas. *Revista Brasileira de Atividade Física e Saúde*, 2, 17-26.

Raso, V., Andrade, E., Matsudo, S., Matsudo, V. (1997). Exercício aeróbico ou de força muscular melhora as variáveis da aptidão física relacionadas a saúde em mulheres idosas. *Revista Brasileira de Atividade Física e Saúde*, 2, 36-49.

Raso, V., Matsudo, S., Matsudo, V., Andrade, E. (1997). Efeito de três protocolos de treinamento na aptidão física de mulheres idosas. *Gerontologia*, 5, 162-170.

Silva, A., Matsudo, S., Matsudo, V. (1999). Efeitos de um programa de ginástica localizada nas variáveis de aptidão física em senhoras acima de 50 anos. In: *Anais XXII Simpósio Internacional de Ciências do Esporte* (pp. 127); 1999 Oct. 7-10. São Paulo, Brasil: Celafiscs.

World Health Organization. (1997). *The World Health Report 1997*. Geneva: WHO.

Non-Specialist Bibliography

Heikkinen, R. (1998). *The role of physical activity in healthy ageing*. Geneva: World Health Organization.

Governo Do Estado De São Paulo. (1998). Secretaria de Estado da Saúde. *Programa Agita São Paulo*. São Paulo.

Matsudo, S., Matsudo, V. (1992). Prescrição e benefícios da atividade física na terceira idade. *Revista Brasileira de Ciência e Movimento*, 6, 19-30.

National Institute On Ageing. (1999). *Exercise: A guide from the National Institute on Ageing*. Gaithersburg.

World Health Organization. (1999). *Ageing: exploding the myths*. Geneva: WHO.

World Health Organization. (1996). WHO Guidelines for physical activity in older persons. *Fouth International Congress of Physical Activity, Ageing and Sports*; 1996. August 27-31; Heidelberg, Germany: University of Heidelberg.

World Health Organization. (1989). *Growth of the elderly population of the world*. Geneva: (WHO – Technical Report Series, 779).

Specialist Bibliography

Berg, W., Lapp, B. (1998). The effect of a practical resistance training intervention on mobility in independent, community-dwelling older adults. *Journal of Ageing and Physical Activity*, 6,18-35.

Evans, W. (1999). Exercise training guidelines for the elderly. *Medicine and Science in Sport and Exercise,* 31, 12-17.

Fiatarone, M. (1996). Physical activity and functional independence in ageing. *Research Quarterly in Exercise and Sport*, 6, 70.

Fiatarone, M., Marks, E., Ryan, N. (1990). High-intensity strength training in nonagenarians: effects on skeletal muscle. *Journal of the American Medical Association,* 263, 3029-3034.

Hurley, B., Hagberg, J. (1998). Optimizing health in older persons: aerobic or strength training? Exercise and Sport Science Reviews, 26, 61-90.

King, A., Rejeski, W., Buchner, D. (1998). Physical activity interventions targeting older adults. A critical review and recommendations. *American Journal of Preventive Medicine*, 15, 316-333.

Lan, C., Lai, J., Chen, S., Wong, M. (1998). 12-month Tai Chi training in the elderly: Its effect on health fitness. *Medicine and Science in Sport and Exercise*, 30, 345-351.

Layne, J., Nelson, M. (1999). The effects of progressive resistance training on bone density: a review. *Medicine and Science in Sport and Exercise*, 31, 25-30.

Rikli, R., Jones, J. (1999). Development and validation of a functional fitness test for community-residing older adults. *Journal of Physical Activity and Ageing, 7,* 129-161.

Spirduso, W. (1995). *Physical Dimensions of Ageing.* Champaign, IL: Human Kinetics.

Wannamethee, G., Shaper, G., Walker, M. (1998). Physical activity alterations, mortality and coronary disease prevalence in older men. *Lancet,* 351, 1603-8.

Wood, R., Reyes-Alvarez, R., Maraj, B., Metoyer, K., Welsch, M. (1999). Physical fitness, cognitive function, and health-related quality of life in older adults. *Journal of Ageing and Physical Activity, 7,* 217-230.

Yan, J., Downing, J. (1998). Tai Chi: an alternative exercise form for seniors. *Journal of Ageing and Physical Activity,* 6, 350-362.

Yan, J. (1998). Tai Chi practice improves senior citizens' balance and arm movement control. *Journal of Ageing and Physical Activity,* 6, 271-284.

Young, D., Appel, L., Jee, S., Miller, E. (1999). The effects of aerobic exercise and T'ai Chi on blood pressure in older people: results of a randomized trial. *Journal of the American Geriatric Society,* 47, 277-284.

Internet

Agita São Paulo Program - Brazil
<www.agitasp.com.br>
E-mail: agitasp@celafics.com.br

Muevete Bogota – Columbia
<www. idrd.gov.co>
E-mail: muevetebogota@usa.net

Participaction – Canada
<www.participaction.com>

Ageing/Health – World Health Organization
<www.who.int/ageing/global_movement>
E-mail: activeageing@who.ch

"Motivated Ageing"
The Perspective of Sports Educational Gerontology

Michael Kolb

Introduction

The phenomenon of a far-reaching demographic shift, or rather of demographic ageing in the entire population is unique in the history of man and has consequences for social development that can hardly be imagined and has become more and more the centre of public attention. The problem is that the focus of the discussion lies primarily on the critical aspects which go hand in hand with ageing, such as on the economic safeguarding of ageing and its social financing.

Similar to the debate about the preventive effects of physical activity, it seems that in this context a new strategy of legitimisation in sport science is going to be established which states that negative physical and mental ageing processes can be slowed down by physical activity. The question remains, however, whether the impression caused by social problems influences the way goals are set. These goals, which are put in the forefront may be seen critically as foundation stones for sport for the elderly. Recommendations for intervention always explicitly or implicitly contain ideas of a desirable final state. It was always an important goal of pedagogic thinking to reflect such objectives. Therefore, the task of sports educational gerontology (see Kolb, 1999; Knowles, 1984; Knowles, 1968)[1]

---

[1] The German terms "Andragogik", which refers to the education of adults, and "Geragogik", which refers to the education of elderly, both were formed in analogy to pedagogy. Meanwhile they are established terms in the educational sciences in Germany. The term "Sportgeragogik" was first used by Meusel (1976, p. 275) and in the following is translated as sports educational gerontology.

Correspondence to: Dr. Michael Kolb, Institut für Sportwissenschaften, Abteilung Sportpädagogik, Universität Wien, Auf der Schmelz 6a, 1150 Wien, Austria.

is to show which normative images form the basis of certain models for sport for the elderly. Furthermore, sports educational gerontologists have to find out about the life standards that confront the elderly and they have to draw up convenient objectives.

In the following text current dominant models and theoretical reasons for sport for the elderly are presented and critical aspects which are part of this argumentation are highlighted. The main focus of this chapter lies on gerontology and educational gerontology: two unique sciences which deal with age and ageing. The special life situation of the elderly in our modern individualised societies is presented and the special requirements are emphasised which contribute to successful ageing. Finally, the objectives and perspectives which are derived from this knowledge, and which form the basis for well-founded sport for the elderly, are pointed out.

Models and Objectives of Sport for the Elderly

If one contemplates the sport science literature about sport for the elderly, one finds two basic models. Either "the sport stereotype is subordinated to the age stereotype or the characteristics of the age are adapted to the standardisation of performance, competition and success, which are connected to the sport image" (Müller, 1986, p. 15). On the one hand there is *sport* for the elderly in which an often life-long athletic career is continued and in which age plays a minor role. On the other hand there is a model of sport for the *elderly* which is in the centre of further analysis. The recommended physical activities aim at fighting the negative effects of ageing and levelling out the processes of degeneration. Sport is subordinated to preventative and therapeutic objectives and the physical demands are adapted to the reduced physical capabilities of the elderly. The central focus is the "preservation of the physical capability and the reduction of the consequences of the natural ageing process in the sense of health prevention or of a sport activity therapy" (Meusel, 1982, p. 23). The physical activities are aimed at optimal preservation, especially of the motor functions, but also of the psychological and social functions.

In particular, the research results of sports medicine show that an intervention in the ageing process using physical training is possible. The performance of metabolism, the function of the single organs, as well as the ability to adapt to physical activities is reduced during the ageing process, but sports medicine research has proven a high development capacity for physical functions even up to an old age (Weineck, 1994, p. 346 ff.; Meusel 1996, p. 41 f.).

According to Lang (1975, p. 76) "the course of the cardiopulmonary functions of the elderly is very similar to the course of people who are sedentary". The result that a lack of physical activity causes similar bodily degeneration as the process of ageing is the decisive theoretical reason for sport for the elderly (compare Badtke & Israel 1985, p. 532; Spirduso, 1995). Often the conviction is taken that "age atrophy is not only a purely regressive biological phenomenon, but a more or less clearly differentiated recessive adaptation process to the reduction of physical activity of the elderly" (compare Lang & Lang 1993, p. 430; Evans, 1998; German & Fried, 1989; Hazzard, 1997). Thus, one presumes that the reduction of the physical function capability of the elderly is due to two reasons. The degeneration which is due to too little activity can be avoided or at least "reduced" according to the results of a training program which was carried out with older people (Lang & Lang, 1990, p. 139; ACSM, 1998; King et al., 1998).

At the same time one presumes that the preservation of physical functions and of physical capability are fundamental prerequisites for satisfying life in old age. Thus according to Lang and Lang (1990, p. 145; Rowe & Kahn, 1987; Hazzard, 1997; Fried et al., 1997) "physical activity even in old age leads to an improvement of mobility, of physical capability, of the capability to cope with stress, and thus to an improvement of life quality". This picture of physical fitness as an essential prerequisite for quality of life in old age is represented over and over again. According to Kirchner (1997, p. 184) quality of life depends "mainly on the level of the individual motor capability and skill capability". The preservation of physical fitness is the fundamental objective of sport for the elderly because "sufficient physical activity is of great importance for a high quality of life" (Meusel, 1996, p. XI).

This argument mainly contains a compensatory idea (compare Beckers & Mayer, 1991, p. 54; Allmer & Tokarski et al., 1996, p. 5). The compensatory reduction of negative ageing processes is the main task of sport for the elderly. According to a perspective focusing on performance, a life model moves to the centre of attention in which the advancement to "the age of highest performance" is followed by an unavoidable degeneration process. In view of the physical capability, the general task is, at most, to slow down the degenerating phase.

Critical Aspects of Function-Orientated Compensatory Sport for the Elderly

From a sports medical point of view, there is proof that the human body can be trained up until old age, and that physical capability can be improved in such a way that it is similar to that of a considerably younger person. The influence of training on the physical ageing process is still unknown. It is not clear yet if a reduction of physical capability in old age can be countered by training or if this burdens the adaptation reserves so heavily that it results in a reduction of the capability to compensate for physical stress. Such an interpretation is suggested by Mader's research results about cellular mechanisms of training adaptation (see 1990 and Mader & Ullmer, 1995; Evans, 1998; Hazzard et al., 1994). Mader presumes that there is a flowing balance between protein decomposition and protein synthesis in the cell; whereas the rate of the protein decomposition determines the genetic transcription activity and thus the production of new protein. If there is a reduced or an increased functional demand, e.g. because of physical repose or physical stress, the reduced or intensified wear and tear of protein reduces or stimulates the transcription activity to produce new protein, which is also called "protein turnover". Here it is important to note that this process cannot be optionally increased, but that there is only a limited adaptation reserve in the sense of a saturation of the protein synthesis.

Danner and Schröder (see 1992, p. 101) point out that studies about the mechanisms of biological ageing have found a general slowing down of the RNA - and the protein - metabolism. According to Mader and Ullmer (1995, p. 40 ff.; Hazzard, 1994; Goldstein, 1993) the consequences are that the protein turnover for the preservation of the total mass is clearly increased and that the function reserve is gradually exhausted when the capacity for the protein production is reduced. If additionally a functional strain of training is present, then there is the danger especially for people of old age, that strains which cannot be compensated become too high. This leads to the question of whether the apparent positive health effects in the sense of improved physical fitness are gained at the expense of stress and at the expense of a "possible wear and tear of regenerative structures of the organism, such as the genes" (Mader & Ullmer, 1995, p. 49; Goldstein, 1993).

The idea of compensation also poses another problem. Here one implicitly thinks only of a body which functions perfectly. Accordingly, the ageing process looks like a degenerative process which goes hand in hand with illnesses and increasing functional disturbances. One derives a necessary fight against ageing processes from the parallelism of health and physical capability, and the parallelism of illness and old age. "Successful" ageing is characterised by good physical fitness (Rowe & Kahn, 1987; Hazzard, 1997; Fried et al., 1997). Insufficient fitness must lead to a concept of dissatisfying and problematic ageing.

Such a concept of sport for the elderly implicitly contains the idea that only a body which functions well can give rise to a "satisfying" old age and a good quality of life. Thus the strange paradox arises that it is the goal of ageing not to get older. Or as Dittmann-Kohli (1989, p. 306) puts it: "Successful ageing is not ageing." Nevertheless, the question is if it is a convenient goal of ageing not to get older and if it is convenient to maintain the physical capability of mid-life as long as possible. Thus, sport for the elderly becomes sport against ageing although its aim would be better in providing support for successful ageing.

Altogether it must be critically seen that the preservation of physical ability in connection with the ageing process is highly emphasised. Whether such a clear connection exists can be doubted according to gerontological knowledge. Recently, the Berlin Elderly Research Project has proved that according to earlier studies, there is no clear connection between an objective physical state and an individual feeling of well-being. However, the subjective judgement of one's life as well as the positive judgement of one's health, along with the contentedness with one's financial situation, with one's social relations and one's participation in social life, are all far more important for general well-being than the state of one's health according to medical criteria (Smith et al., 1996; Antonocci & Akiyama, 1987; Kastenbaum, 1995; Martin et al., 1992; Poon et al., 1992).

The danger of a functional orientation of sport for the elderly is that the usual notions of one's own physical capability are confirmed and that the elderly use physical activities to deny their individual inevitable ageing. Furthermore, the idea can arise that one can escape from the negatively marked ageing process by following certain rules for physical activity. If one only tries to deny the ageing process and to repress the losses which go hand in hand with ageing, the consequences are "not only the denial of the human condition, but also the repression of new possibilities for development" (Kruse, 1988, p. 475). Here old age is not seen as an independent life period, but rather as a stage which must be avoided for as long as possible.

It is also a problem that a positive image brings along a negative image as well. All those who do not fit, and who do not want to fit, into the given picture of a fit and capable elderly person are ostracised and judged negatively. The result is a contrast between capable ageing, which is reached through physical activity, and negative old age, which is marked by degeneration processes and illnesses. Elderly people who are not physically active and thus do not care for their health, seem to have to justify the negative consequences more and more.

Age gets into a medical-economical discussion which interprets old age as an illness process and a cost factor. The suggestions to participate in sporting activities are thus automatically combined with the social expectations of ageing that it does not bring any costs. Some people already see a "sprightliness competition" (Gronemeyer, 1987, p. 916) in which one demonstrates one's physical capacity in direct comparison to others. Thus, sport for the elderly is in danger of becoming part of the many cosmetic and preventive efforts to hide one's ageing from of others and finally from oneself as well.

These critical remarks certainly do not mean that sport should not be used for the elderly to fight physical degeneration processes. Nevertheless, sport for the elderly has to be classed in a reasonable educational gerontological concept which does not raise the idea that the ageing process can be handled by a training programme. Rather, it should emphasise the special requirements and opportunities which are characteristic of the life period of older people.

The Situation and Requirements of the Elderly in Our Modern Societies

The order of single life periods, and the life period of old age itself, are social constructs. The comparatively new life concept of the life stage 'old age' developed in the modern industrial countries in the course of the last one hundred years because of the enormous lengthening of the lifespan and the liberation from work and family obligations (Hudson, 1997).

Traditional social forms and "everyday life cultures" are increasingly dissolved in the process of modernisation. Life does not run in given tracks any longer. Biographies are mainly self-determined on one's own responsibility; they have to be put together and they have to be justified. The social state conditions in particular, such as the educational system and the financing of pensions, force people to make decisions. Biographical choices are often not made voluntarily, but are forced, such as retirement. Therefore, individualisation in the sense of an obligation to plan one's own life in modern societies demands a great deal of skill in biographical self-reflection and the ability to plan life on one's own.

The tendency toward individualisation is valid for the elderly as well and forces them to find their own solutions for the rest of their life after a long history of working or after the maintenance of a certain role in family. According to Langehennig (1987, p. 147) "the way of living and the understanding of life of the people who are ageing now is marked by the obligation to 'biographise' the 'gained years'". Nowadays the old age period is stretched over a comparatively long period of time. This life period which starts after the end of middle age can hardly be lived according to the model of permanent leisure time, but older people need their "own goals and biographical projects" (Kohli et al., 1989, p. 244; Kastenbaum, 1995) to conveniently handle the possibilities of the coming years of their lives. This life period, which is largely liberated from social obligations, as well as the dissolution of age-specific norms for behaviour offer the elderly new options for acting. But at the same time they are left on their own and are forced to construct their life according to their own standards. The central task is to construct a personal and reasonable perspective for the rest of one's life. But the liberation of life-structuring tasks, the loss of many important personal sources which gave life meaning, the accumulation of critical events, and the little time that is left for living are conditions which make this more difficult.

Therefore, a picture of successful ageing which is valid for all human beings cannot exist. Only individual forms of successful ageing are possible which, according to biographies, personal life goals and existing life possibilities, can be of completely different character. With regard to this image of modern societies, nobody can put up normative models of how the last life period best can be mastered. Therefore, in the course of its development gerontology has dissociated itself more and more from the draft of normative pictures of successful ageing. It is not of great importance that a certain level of activities or the preservation of certain physical capabilities are maintained, but it is important that the individual succeeds in finding his personal life perspectives and can orient his life accordingly in spite of the difficult life changes.

The ability to newly orient oneself and to structure old age through a revision of previous goals and preferences is of great importance because old age is marked by breaks, critical life events, and transitions. Featherman (1989, p. 11) talks of a special "competence for adaptation" which he classifies as an ability "to react with adaptation to the challenge of unpredictable changes of the little structured life situation". Rosenmayr (1994, p. 168) talks of a "discontinuity ability" or a "handling of life with flexibility" (Rosenmayr, 1990, p. 96) in which external changes are answered by one's own changing processes (see also Hirsch & Hirsch, 1998).

The existence of abilities which are necessary for self-development in old age can hardly be expected from older people. According to previous results of gerontology, these abilities depend on the individual biography, especially educational background, social status, the kind of job, and socio-economic situation (Baecker & Naegele, 1993, p. 140). Therefore, the central question of education for the elderly is how older people can be motivated to find out about new perspectives with regard to the world and to themselves, and how they can be enabled to find personal life goals even under unfavourable life conditions. The centre of attention of education for the elderly does not have to lie only on the preservation and compensation of abilities. Instead, old age has to be presented as being an independent life period. The awareness of the range of possible life- and value-orientations must be raised and older people's readiness to think over and to revise previous goals and previous behaviour needs to be strengthened. Such an education for the elderly aims for "emancipated old age" in which older people are supported in the best way possible to decide for themselves how they want to get older (Fried et al., 1997).

Perspectives of Sports Educational Gerontology

The relevant question within sports educational gerontology is the contribution to successful ageing made by sporting activities and games. It is convenient for legitimated sport for the elderly to orient itself using higher education goals, such as: personal flexibility, an opportunity for new experiences, a reflection of one's life and an outline of new life perspectives. These goals cannot simply be reached through the instruction to do sporting activities.

Already Rosenmayr (1981, p. 25) has criticised this idea which is similar to the gerontological activity theory: "To be active and to be able to change oneself is not the same thing at all. Activity is only one of many conditions for a developmental ability in old age. On the contrary: change requires reflection and thus distance and an activity break. Activity can be an unconscious defensive strategy to avoid necessary changes." From this perspective sporting activities in old age should be treated as an integral part of a general education process, in which not only self-responsible management of personal sporting activity is suggested, but where development of the individual is initiated beyond the narrow area of the sporting activity. The point is to sensitise the elderly for a changed perception of the individual and the social environment; broaden habitual perspectives; discover possibilities which enrich life; and establish flexibility for the management of old age (Hirsch & Hirsch, 1998).

The goal of sport for the elderly is in various ways "Motivated Ageing" in the sense of supporting older people with the help of sporting activities to experience the last phase of life, old age, in a way that is worthwhile and constructive. In this respect, sport education in old age has to offer room for action in which personal and social experiences can be made. In contrast to the model of sport for the elderly which tries to secure physical continuity through training programmes, it is preferable to create situations which demand different actions so that the older participants can experience success in various sporting activities despite some limitations. Thus these activities can lead to a feeling openness to different types of exercise experiences. There are hardly any didactic approaches to such an educational orientation to sport for the elderly. Nevertheless, it seems to be important that the elderly get opportunities of every kind to be active, creative, engaged in activities and in contact with one another. The experience that different situations can be handled in many ways can be provided by offering sporting activities which contain a concentrated perception of their own body, diverse social contact, as well as games and movement tasks. This perspective contains the hope that the experience which is gained through involvement in certain situations leads to greater openness and flexibility in the individual's personality which is reflected by overcoming conscious preoccupation with ageing. A fundamental goal is to accept the changes in one's body which are due to ageing. The realistic acceptance of physical changes, as well as the development of a physical sensibility which perhaps had not been experienced yet, is of great importance.

Well-balanced sport education for the elderly should have the goal of maintaining physical fitness, accepting losses due to ageing, as well as distancing oneself from the previous picture of one's own body. "Natural ageing is only possible with such a 'wise' attitude which accepts remaining abilities, but which realistically judges limited competence as well" (Minnemann, 1994, p. 144; Poon et al., 1992).

Acknowledgement:

With special thanks to Dr. Mark Alexander Hirsch[2] for contributing the English literature resources and constructive comments to this text.

---

[2] Dr. Mark A. Hirsch, Wilhelm-Tell-Str. 27, 40219 Düsseldorf, Germany. E-mail: park20@hotmail.com

References

Allmer, H. & Tokarski, W. u. a. (1996). *Bewegung, Spiel und Sport im Alter. Band II: Strukturelle Merkmale von Angeboten.* Köln: Sport und Buch Strauß.

American College of Sports Medicine Position Stand. (1998). Exercise and physical activity for older adults. *Medicine and Science in Sports and Exercise,* 53(10), 46, 49-52, 61-62.

Antonucci, T., & Akiyama, H. (1987). Social networks in adult life and a preliminary examination of the convoy model. *Journal of Gerontology,* 42, 519-527.

Badtke, G. & Israel, S. (1985). Sportliche Belastbarkeit im höheren Lebensalter. *Wissenschaftliche Zeitschrift der Pädagogischen Hochschule Potsdam,* 29, 527-537.

Baecker, G. & Naegele, G. (1993). Geht die Entberuflichung zu Ende? Perspektiven einer Neuorganisation der Alterserwerbsarbeit. In Naegele, G. & Tews, H.P. (Hrsg.), *Lebenslagen im Strukturwandel des Alters. Alternde Gesellschaft - Folgen für die Politik* (135-157). Opladen: Westdeutscher Verlag.

Beck, U. (1986). *Risikogesellschaft. Auf dem Weg in eine andere Moderne.* Frankfurt: Suhrkamp.

Beckers, E. & Mayer, M. (1991). Jugendliches Altern. Zur Ambivalenz von Altern und Bewegen. *Brennpunkte der Sportwissenschaft,* 5 (1), 50-74.

Bringmann, W. (1982). Sport im höheren Lebensalter. *Zeitschrift für Alternsforschung,* 37, 391-399.

Danner, D.B. & Schröder, H.C. (1992). Biologie des Alterns (Ontogenese und Evolution). In P.B. Baltes & J. Mittelstaß (Hrsg.), *Zukunft des Alterns und gesellschaftliche Entwicklung. Akademie der Wissenschaften zu Berlin. Forschungsbericht 5* (95-123). Berlin, New York: Walter de Gruyter.

Dittmann-Kohli, F. (1989). Erfolgreiches Altern aus subjektiver Sicht. In P.B. Baltes, M. Kohli, & K. Sames (Hrsg.), *Erfolgreiches Altern. Bedingungen und Variationen* (S. 301-307). Bern, Stuttgart, Toronto, Seattle: Hans Huber.

Evans, W.J. (1998). Exercise and nutritional needs of elderly people: effects on muscle and bone. *Gerontology*, 15(1), 15-24.

Featherman, D.L. (1989). Erfolgreiches Altern: Adaptive Kompetenz in einer Ruhestandsgesellschaft. In P.B. Baltes, M. Kohli, & K. Sames (Hrsg.), Erfolgreiches Altern. *Bedingungen und Variationen* (S. 11-18). Bern, Stuttgart, Toronto, Seattle: Hans Huber.

Fried, L.P., Freedman, M., Endres, T.E., & Wasik, B . (1997). Building communities that promote successful aging. *Western Journal of Medicine,* 167(4), 216-219.

German, P.S., & Fried, L.P. (1989). Prevention and the elderly: Public health issues and strategies. *Annual Review of Public Health*, 26, 61-89.

Goldstein, S. (1993). The biology of aging: Looking to defuse the genetic time bomb. *Geriatrics*, 48(9), 76-82.

Gronemeyer, M. (1987). *Altwerden - Aufbruch und Abschied*. Universitas, 42, 913-922.

Hazzard, W.R. (1997). Ways to make "usual" and "successful" aging synonymous: preventive gerontology. In: *Successful Aging, Westernal Journal of Medicine*, 167, 206-215.

Hazzard, W.R., Andres, R., Bierman, E.L., & Blass, J.P. (Eds.). (1994). *Principles of Geriatric Medicine and Gerontology, 3rd edition*. New York: McGraw-Hill.

Hirsch, M.A. & Hirsch, H.V.B. (1998). Novel activities enhance performance of the aging brain. *Journal of Physical Education Recreation & Dance,* 69(8), 15-19.

Hudson, R.B. (Ed.). (1997). *The Future of Age-Based Public Policy.* Baltimore, Maryland: Johns Hopkins University Press.

Jones, C.J., & Rikli, R.E. (1993). The gerontology movement-Is it passing us by? *Journal of Physical Education Recreation & Dance,* 1, 17-26.

Kastenbaum, R.J. (Ed.). (1995). The Georgia Centenarian Study (Special Issue). *International Journal of Aging and Adult Development,* 41(2).

King, A.C., Rejeski, W.J., & Buchner, D.M. (1998). Physical activity interventions targeting older adults: A critical review and recommendations. *American Journal of Preventive Medicine,* 15(4), 316-333.

Kirchner, G. (1997). Motorisches Lernen im Alter. Ergebnisse, Fragestellungen, Ziele. In H. Baumann & M. Leye (Hrsg)., *Bewegung und Sport mit älteren Menschen. Wie - Was - Warum?* (S. 183-198). Aachen: Meyer & Meyer.

Kirchner, G. & Schaller, H.-J. (1996). *Motorisches Lernen im Alter. Grundlagen und Anwendungsperspektiven.* Aachen: Meyer & Meyer.

Knowles, M.S. (1984). *The adult learner: A neglected species.* (3rd ed.), Houston: Gulf Publishing.

Knowles, M.S. (1968). Androgogy, not pedagogy! *Adult Leadership,* 16, 350-352, 386.

Kohli, M. (1986). Gesellschaftszeit und Lebenszeit. Der Lebenslauf im Strukturwandel der Moderne. In J. Berger (Hrsg.), *Die Moderne - Kontinuität und Zäsuren. Soziale Welt, Sonderband 4,* 183-208.

Kohli, M. u. a. (1989). *Je früher - desto besser? Die Verkürzung des Erwerbslebens am Beispiel des Vorruhestandes in der chemischen Industrie.* Berlin: Rainer Bohn.

Kolb, M. (1999): *Bewegtes Altern. Grundlagen und Perspektiven einer Sportgeragogik.* Schorndorf: Hofmann.

Kolb, M. (1995). *Spiele für den Herz- und Alterssport. Perspektive und Praxis einer spielorientierten Bewegungstherapie. (Schriftenreihe Behinderte machen Sport Bd. 3).* Aachen: Meyer & Meyer.

Kruse, A. (1988). Gerontologische Aspekte und theologische Fragestellungen. In A. Kruse u. a. (Hrsg.), *Gerontologie - Wissenschaftliche Erkenntnisse und Folgerungen für die Praxis. Beiträge zur II. Gerontologischen Woche* (S. 466-500). München: Bayerischer Monatsspiegel Verlagsgesellschaft.

Lang, E. (1975). Sport und präklinische Geriatrie. *Sportarzt und Sportmedizin,* 26 (4), 76-80.

Lang, E. & Lang, B.M. (1993). Bewegung als Prävention vor Krankheit im Alter. *Zeitschrift für Gerontologie,* 26, 429-435.

Lang, E. & Lang, B.M. (1990). Die Bedeutung von körperlicher Aktivität und Sport in den verschiedenen Lebensphasen. In R. Schmitz-Scherzer, A. Kruse & E. Olbrich (Hrsg.), *Altern - Ein lebenslanger Prozeß der sozialen Interaktion* (S. 139-146). Darmstadt: Steinkopff.

Langehennig, M. (1987). *Die Seniorenphase im Lebenslauf: Zur sozialen Konstruktion eines neuen Lebensalters.* Augsburg: Maro.

Mader, A. (1990). Aktive Belastungsadaptation und Regulation der Proteinsynthese auf zellulärer Ebene. *Deutsche Zeitschrift für Sportmedizin,* 41, 40-58.

Mader, A. & Ullmer, S. (1995). Biologische Grundlagen der Trainingsanpassung und der Bezug zu den Begriffen Gesundheit, Fitneß und Alter. In W. Schlicht & P. Schwenkmezger (Hrsg.), *Gesundheitsverhalten und Bewegung* (S. 35-59). Schorndorf: Hofmann.

Martin, P., Poon, L.W., Clayton, G.M., Lee, H.S., Fulks, J.S., & Johnson, M.A. (1992). Personality, life events, and coping in the oldest-old. *International Journal of Aging and Adult Development,* 34(1), 19-30.

Meusel, H. (1996). *Bewegung, Sport und Gesundheit im Alter.* Wiesbaden: Quelle & Meyer.

Meusel, H. (1982). *Sport, Spiel, Gymnastik in der zweiten Lebenshälfte. Ziele, Training, Unterricht, Organisation.* Bad Homburg, Frankfurt am Main: Limpert.

Meusel, H. (1976). *Einführung in die Sportpädagogik.* München: Wilhelm Fink.

Minnemann, E. (1994). *Die Bedeutung sozialer Beziehungen für Lebenszufriedenheit im Alter.* Regensburg: S. Roderer.

Müller, M. (1986). *Alter und/oder Sport.* Zur Dissonanz eines Phänomens. Diss. Marburg.

Poon, L.W., Martin, P., Clayton, G. M., Messner, S., Noble, C.A., & Johnson, M.A. (1992). The influence of cognitive resources on adaptation and old age. *International Journal of Aging and Adult Development,* 34, 31-46.

Rosenmayr, L. (1994). Altersgesellschaft - bunte Gesellschaft? Soziologische Analyse als Beitrag zur politischen Orientierung. *Journal für Sozialforschung,* 34, 145-172.

Rosenmayr, L. (1990). *Die Kräfte des Alters.* Wien: Atelier.

Rosenmayr, L. (1981). Altersvorbereitung - ein Weg zu sich selbst? In Pro Senectute (Hrsg.), *Vorbereitung auf das Alter im Lebenslauf. Beiträge aus Theorie und Praxis* (S. 17-38). Paderborn: Schöningh.

Rowe, J.W., & Kahn, R.L. (1987). Human aging: usual and successful: a review. *Science,* 237, 143-149.

Spirduso, W.W. (1995). *Physical Dimensions of Aging.* Champaign, IL: Human Kinetics.

Smith, J. u. a. (1996). Wohlbefinden im Alter: Vorhersagen aufgrund objektiver Lebensbedingungen und subjektiver Bewertung. In K.-U. Mayer, & P.B. Baltes (Hrsg.), *Die Berliner Altersstudie. Ein Projekt der Berlin-Brandenburgischen Akademie der Wissenschaften* (S. 497-523). Berlin: Akademie.

Weineck, J. (1994). *Sportbiologie (4. Aufl.)*. Erlangen: perimed.

Williamson, J.D., & Fried, L.P. (1996). Characterization of older adults who attribute functional decrements to "old age". *Journal of the American Geriatrics Society*, 44(12), 1429-1434.

Non-Specialist Bibliography - English

Clayton, G.M., Martin, P., Poon, L.W., Lawhorn, L.A., & Avery, K.L. (1993). Survivors. *Nursing and Health Care*, 14(5), 256-260.

Hirsch, M.A. & Hirsch, H.V.B. (1998). Novel activities enhance performance of the aging brain. *Journal of Physical Education Recreation & Dance,* 69(8), 15-19.

Jones, C.J., & Rikli, R.E. (1993). The gerontology movement - Is it passing us by? *Journal of Physical Education Recreation & Dance*, 1, 17-26.

Knowles, M.S. (1984). *The adult learner: A neglected species.* (3rd ed.), Houston: Gulf Publishing.

Spirduso, W.W. (1995). *Physical Dimensions of Aging*. Champaign, IL: Human Kinetics.

Non-Specialist Bibliography – German

Kolb, M. (1995). *Spiele für den Herz- und Alterssport*. Aachen: Meyer & Meyer.

Mertens, K. (Hrsg.) (1997). *Aktivierungs-Programme für Senioren*. Dortmund: Verlag modernes lernen.

Meusel, H. (1999). *Sport für Ältere. Bewegung – Sportarten – Training. Handbuch für Ärzte, Therapeuten, Sportlehrer und Sportler.* Stuttgart, New York: Schattauer.

Meusel, H. (1996). *Bewegung, Sport und Gesundheit im Alter.* Wiesbaden: Quelle & Meyer.

Meusel, H. (1987). *Sport, Spiel, Gymnastik in der zweiten Lebenshälfte. Ziele, Training, Unterricht, Organisation* (2. Aufl.). Bad Homburg, Frankfurt am Main: Limpert.

Philippi-Eisenburger, M. (1991). *Praxis der Bewegungsarbeit mit Älteren.* Schorndorf: Hofmann.

Specialist Bibliography – English

American College of Sports Medicine Position Stand. (1998). Exercise and physical activity for older adults. *Medicine and Science in Sports and Exercise*, 53(10), 46, 49-52, 61-62.

Antonucci, T., & Akiyama, H. (1987). Social networks in adult life and a preliminary examination of the convoy model. *Journal of Gerontology*, 42, 519-527.

Hazzard, W.R. (1997). Ways to make "usual" and "successful" aging synonymous: preventive gerontology. In: *Successful Aging, Westernal Journal of Medicine*, 167, 206-215.

Hazzard, W.R., Andres, R., Bierman, E.L., & Blass, J.P. (Eds.). (1994). *Principles of Geriatric Medicine and Gerontology, 3rd edition.* New York: McGraw-Hill.

Hudson, R.B. (Ed.). (1997). *The Future of Age-Based Public Policy.* Baltimore, Maryland: Johns Hopkins University Press.

Martin, P., Poon, L.W., Clayton, G.M., Lee, H.S., Fulks, J.S., & Johnson, M.A. (1992). Personality, life events, and coping in the oldest-old. *International Journal of Aging and Adult Development*, 34(1), 19-30.

Poon, L.W., Martin, P., Clayton, G.M., Messner, S., Noble, C.A., & Johnson, M.A. (1992). The influence of cognitive resources on adaptation and old age. *International Journal of Aging and Adult Development*, 34, 31-46.

Specialist Bibliography – German

Allmer, H. & Tokarski, W. u. a. (1996). *Bewegung, Spiel und Sport im Alter. Band II: Strukturelle Merkmale von Angeboten.* Köln: Sport und Buch Strauß.

Alterssport (2000). Schwerpunktheft. *Sportwissenschaft*, 29.

Baumann, H. (Hrsg.). (1992). *Altern und körperliches Training.* Bern, Göttingen: Hans Huber.

Baumann, H. & Leye, M. (Hrsg.). (1997*). Bewegung und Sport mit älteren Menschen. Wie - Was - Warum?* Aachen: Meyer & Meyer.

Baur, J. u. a. (1996). *Seniorensport in Ostdeutschland. Zwischen Powersport und Kaffeeklatsch.* Aachen: Meyer & Meyer.

Conzelmann, A. (1997). *Entwicklung konditioneller Fähigkeiten im Erwachsenenalter.* Schorndorf: Hofmann.

Denk, H. (Hrsg.). (1996). *Alterssport. Aktuelle Forschungsergebnisse.* Schorndorf: Hofmann.

Denk, H. & Pache, D. (1996). *Bewegung, Spiel und Sport im Alter. Band I: Bedürfnissituation Älterer.* Köln: Sport und Buch Strauß.

Kolb, M. (2000). „Bewegtes Altern": Perspektiven einer Sportgeragogik. *Sportwissenschaft*, 30, 68-81.

Kolb, M. (1999). *Bewegtes Altern. Grundlagen und Perspektiven einer Sportgeragogik.* Schorndorf: Hofmann.

Mechling, H. (Hrsg.) (1998), *Training im Alterssport. Sportliche Leistungsfähigkeit und Fitness im Alternsprozeß*. Schorndorf: Hofmann.

Philippi-Eisenburger, M. (1990). *Bewegungsarbeit mit älteren und alten Menschen*. Schorndorf: Hofmann.

Winter, R. & Baur, J. (1994). Motorische Entwicklung im Erwachsenenalter. In J. Baur, K. Bös & R. Singer (Hrsg.) *Motorische Entwicklung. Ein Handbuch* (S. 309-332). Schorndorf: Hofmann.

A Physical Activity Programme to Support the Work Ability of Ageing Workers

Characteristics of a Successful Physical Activity Programme

Maaret Ilmarinen

Introduction

Physical functional capacity forms the basis for a person's work ability. Regular physical activity is the only means of maintaining physical functional capacity and resisting the decline in physical, mental and social functional capacity that accelerates with age. Aerobic endurance and muscular fitness decrease as much as 25 % in 5 years after 45 years of age. It is possible, however, for both to be increased by 25 % in the same period if regular physical activity is begun and continued. People who are regularly physically active have been shown to have about 20 functionally capable years more than their sedentary counterparts (Ilmarinen, 1993).

The results of long-term follow-up studies (Ilmarinen, 1993), and questionnaires (Ilmarinen, 1995) on personal perceptions, have shown that physical functional capacity is associated with mental and social work ability. When about 10 000 Finns were asked "How does your leisure-time physical activity affect your physical, mental and social functional ability?", over 75 % responded that physical activity had improved their physical work ability, almost 90 % reported that it had improved their mental work ability, and over 60 % stated that their social work ability had been positively affected (Ilmarinen, 1995). In everyday life, physical activity represents well-being, health, endurance, and quality of life (Laakso et al., 1986). A worker who is physically capable has been found to make the

Correspondence to: Maaret Ilmarinen, M.A., Project Manager Fit for Life Programme, Radiokatu 20, 00240 Helsinki, Finland most of many of the characteristics that develop through long-term work experience. For example, a strategic thought process, sharp intellect, consideration, wisdom, ability to think, control of life, comprehensive perception, controlled use of language, high motivation to learn, work commitment, loyalty towards one's employer, low levels of sick leave, and work experience (Ruoppila, 1996).

For an enterprise, employees with a high functional capacity represent results, productivity, ability to compete and notable savings that can be seen, above all, in statistics on premature retirement, sickness absence, occupational health care expenses and work productivity (Shephard, 1990). For example, Fundia Wire Oy, an enterprise with over 800 workers, invested 0.3 million Finnish marks a year in a physical activity programme and earned 3 million Finnish marks in return, of which 1.6 million marks came from work disability funds, 1.3 million marks from an increase in productivity, and 0.2 million marks from a decrease in sickness absence (Näsman, 1996). ABB, located in Vaasa, was able to decrease the costs of five workers' sickness absence by 190 000 Finnish marks a year (143 workdays) by providing rehabilitation in the form of a personal physical activity programme for workers suffering from musculoskeletal disorders (Manninen, 1996). When a physical activity programme is started for an enterprise, the economic savings are the result of sedentary workers becoming active.

There is also an economic advantage for a society if its population has a high functional capacity. If the average retirement age of the Finnish population could be increased by one year, from 59 to 60, the savings in retirement costs would be about 7 million Finnish marks a year. The current costs of sickness and accidents are over 20 % of the gross national product (i.e. 110 billion Finnish marks a year). When the number of retirees, who are the primary consumers of health care services, doubles in the near future, will the costs of health care also double? Regular physical activity has been proved effective both as a form of prevention and as a form of treatment for many common illnesses, for example, cardiovascular diseases, musculoskeletal diseases, metabolic disorders and mental diseases. Even though using physical activity in the treatment and prevention of these diseases is effective and economical, it has not been used enough for this purpose thus far. The institutional care or treatment of one patient costs society 400,000 Finnish marks per year. Musculoskeletal diseases account for 9 billion marks of this amount (Ahonen, 1995, Vuori, 1996).

The maintenance of one's own functional capacity and health belongs primarily to the person him- or herself. The significance of physical activity, not only to the individual, but also to the work community and society, especially an ageing society, is so great that integrating physical activity into the normal functioning of the work community is justified. This integration should also show in the functional strategy of enterprises. In practice, therefore, each employer should have its own activity programme that motivates, makes possible, and supports the regular activity of personnel.

Characteristics of a Successful Physical Activity Programme

The data presented on the characteristics of successful physical activity programmes in this article are based on the results obtained so far in a 5-year Finnish programme called Fitness for All Ages, which ended in 1999, and also on literature concerning physical activity programmes in employment. The objective of the national Fitness for All Ages programme is to motivate 150 000 sedentary middle-aged persons (40-60 years of age) to join the ranks of the physically active. The programme has 400 local projects, primarily in different types of workplaces, in progress. The local projects keep a record of their activities. The records are then gathered into an annual report at the end of each year. At the end of the project a complete analysis of the data will be made. The following observations are based on the characteristics of projects that have been successful.

A health promotion programme with a good outcome has been achieved when the programme has had the following characteristics: 1) valid justification for initiating the programme, 2) commitment of all factions of the work community, 3) clear aim for change, 4) specific services, 5) available service chains, 6) functional network of co-operation, 7) effective means of promotion, 8) knowledgeable experts able to support the individual worker's changes in life-style, and 9) follow-up and related post-project activity (Ilmarinen, 1998).

For the programme to succeed it must be justified; in other words, there must be good reasons for initiating the project. Some of the arguments for the programme have been described in the preceding section with respect to the individual worker, the work community and society.

Even though a high level of functional capacity creates the basis for productive work, integrating a physical activity programme into other activities to promote work ability - the development of the worker, the work, work conditions, and the work community as a whole - remains important.

Commitment of the Work Community

The success of an activity programme depends on the commitment of the different sectors of the work community. Thus management, immediate supervisors and foremen, and the entire work force must be convinced that the programme has significance. Especially important are the commitment and enthusiasm of key persons, which, in the end, make the difference between success or failure. Commitment requires information about the significance of physical activity and its possibilities, but positive personal experiences with physical activity are also often valuable. Being able to promote the significance of physical activity to workers and the workplace as a whole in an understandable and interesting manner is essential.

The programme can be promoted as part of the strategy for personnel training and communication; it can be directed partially toward the entire work force and partially toward specific target groups. In making choices as to how to promote the programme and develop commitment, it is essential to differentiate between the motives of the individual workers and those of enterprises and society as a whole. People as individuals are known to be motivated by the fact that physical activity can provide fitness and a good appearance, health, stimulating experiences, possibilities for recreation and relaxation, the company of friends and nature, an opportunity to express themselves, the excitement brought on by physical effort, competition, the joy of learning, and feelings of endurance and well-being (Laakso et al. 1986; see also other references in this report). The management and supervisors of a firm are ready to initiate and support a physical activity programme if they are aware of the way it can affect productivity, savings, the perseverance and health of the work force, and the work atmosphere. Municipal decision makers are naturally interested in the savings produced by physical activity programmes; such savings can especially be seen in social and health care costs and also in the costs of retirement benefits (Ahonen, 1995; Bergström, 1997).

The commitment of decision makers may not only depend on their being given access to available information and data; they may also need more personal means of familiarising themselves with the possibilities, through a pilot project, for example.

The commitment of the entire work force is also promoted by the possibility of the programme being carried out partially on work time. There are many ways to do this, for example, an hour a week of physical activity on work time, fitness tests during work time, sports days, special excursions, the commute to work in a physically active form partially being counted as work time, "walking" meetings, daily exercises during a work break, exercise breaks for specific work sites or stations.

Decision and Objectives

Once the different sectors of the work community become convinced of the significance of the physical activity programme, a decision is needed to initiate the programme and establish its goals. The workers with a poor level of fitness and functional capacity will benefit the most from such a programme. Increasing this group's work ability is also the most beneficial for both the work community as a whole and also society. Therefore, activating the sedentary members of the work force to participate in regular physical activity is the most important goal, and the success of this task is, in the end, determined by the results of the project. It would also be of use to select the objectives of the programme with this fact in mind. The goals can also emphasise the activation of older workers, who can be motivated through special measures involving follow-up or rewards. In addition, the importance of some activity in place of a completely passive life-style can be emphasised, and every instance of physical activity can be taken into consideration no matter what the frequency or duration. It is important that the objectives of the programme be simple and clear. If so, making the needed commitment is easy, and progress towards fulfilment can be followed.

The following goals are suitable as general objectives of the programme:

1) to increase and maintain the regular activity, fitness and functional capacity of personnel;
2) to support personnel's ability to cope and relax;
3) to improve the work atmosphere;
4) to insure the overall productivity of the work community.

These objectives can be attained, for example, through the following respective actions:
5) increasing the proportion of workers who are regularly physically active, increasing the personal results of the workers on the fitness tests so that the minimum fitness level is average or the workers' weight and other measurements (waist, hip, etc.) decrease either on an individual basis or as a group;
6) finding a suitable form of activity for every worker, a relaxing or refreshing hobby or physical activity in natural surroundings;
7) initiating a joint form of physical activity for management, supervisors and workers (general physical activity services for the entire work community, combined sports days, competitions between departments, etc.);
8) decreasing sickness absence, improving productivity, and decreasing premature retirement.

Success with either a Limited or Broad Programme

The physical activity objective can be reached in many ways and with different amounts of investment. A limited programme can be realised, for example, through an annual fitness card campaign in which the actual programme remains completely in the hands of the worker. The enterprise merely rewards the personnel who have been sufficiently active or groups or departments which have recruited new participants. A broad programme can include sections in which the different interest groups of the workplace such as: management, personnel administrators, occupational health care professionals, safety officers, and chosen worker representatives, receive education that helps them to plan and run the programme and also carry out any testing that is needed. The activity is planned on the basis of a workplace-related analysis, responses to questionnaires, and the results of tests. On the basis of their fitness, symptoms and interests, the workers are offered a diverse range of physical activity either entirely or partly carried out at the expense of the enterprise and partly on work time. The progress of the programme is followed with the aid of different measures, which are directed towards the workplace as a whole, towards the departments and also towards the individual workers. The programme is then updated according to the results of the tests and analyses. The enterprise can carry out the programme through the aid of its own personnel as a part of its programme to maintain the work ability of its workers or it can purchase part or all of the services needed.

Numerous alternatives can be found between the simplest and broadest forms of programmes. Sometimes good results can be obtained with very small input, but there is no reason to avoid large investments either because research has shown that the return to the enterprise from physical activity programmes can be double or even five times the costs (Shephard, 1990). Whether the programme is carried out in a limited or broad form, it should be remembered that good results always require long-term commitment, preferably a permanent one. Short-term campaigns have not proved to be of any benefit; instead they represent the squandering of resources.

Specific Services

Specific services take into consideration the needs and desires of the individual workers. It is important to listen to the comments of all parties, but emphasis should nevertheless be on sedentary workers. The workplace can create its own strategy for people who are regularly active, those who are irregularly active, and also for those who are beginners. Different forms of introductory courses and an easy means of following fitness should be offered to the beginners. The physical activity can also be planned to fit the demands of the work, whether it be physically or mentally stressful, and according to typical symptoms of workers, for example, groups for people with musculoskeletal, back or weight problems or such symptoms as anxiety, depression or burnout. It is especially important that workers with a heavy physical work load and repetitive and monotonous movements be taken into consideration in that they need stimulating and relaxing activity in place of physical strain. Physical activity for workers with heavy work loads demands special skill and instruction.

Service Chain for Health-Related Physical Activities

The allocation of services and the continuation of a physical activity programme can, once begun, be strengthened by a continuum of special services (Table 1). The chain should offer services for beginners with different levels of fitness and also alternatives for them to continue in new groups that are challenging and interesting. The service network should also slowly shift the emphasis from instruction to self-activity. It is important, however, that the activity levels of the workers be followed continually as a part of enterprise or occupational health activity.

Service Provided	Service Provider
Prescription for physical activity (follow-up, fitness testing, examinations)	Occupational health care unit
Rehabilitative group activity	Rehabilitation unit of a health care service, occupational physiotherapist, occupational health nurse
Group activity for beginners	Physical activity director, civic college or institute, physical activity instructor at the workplace
Other types of physical activity	Municipalities, sports club, private physical activity services, self-directed physical activity
Constant follow-up, meetings for feedback	Health care services, client registers of occupational health units, fitness tests

Table 1. Service chain for physical activity to maintain work ability

Functional Network of Co-operation

The possibility of establishing a versatile and economic programme is greater if co-operation is developed with other organisations, especially in the case of small and middle-sized enterprises. The local producers of physical activity services and also other organisations needing physical activity services are important partners. The more important producers of physical activity services are the municipal sports and recreation offices, sports clubs, social and health associations, civic schools and institutes, and pertinent private enterprises. In addition, sports institutes, regional sections of sports and physical activity associations, and provincial sports and recreation boards work with health-related physical activity. Other organisations needing physical activity services are, of course, other workplaces in the same area. An example of some good local networks are presented in a later section of this paper.

Effective Promotion

The success of an enterprise's physical activity programme not only depends on the information activities referred to in the discussion on commitment later in this paper. For the results to be favourable, knowledge is needed on how the physical activity programme will be carried out, and specific information on the contents, events and services to be offered must be available.

The experts participating in the execution of the programme (physicians, health nurses, physiotherapists, and physical activity instructors) should be knowledgeable about the effects of physical activity on health and also about proper dosages of physical activity for the relevant age grouping. Sometimes these data interest the participants as well. The more important questions are how different types of physical activity behaviour and different forms of physical activity affect different health factors, how adults or elderly persons should begin regular physical activities, what amount and intensity of physical activity should be used for workers with different fitness and skill levels, and what forms of activity suit beginners. Much data on these questions can be found in the literature (e.g., Vuori, 1996; Louhevaara & Smolander 1996).

The specific information on the physical activity programme is directly connected with the content of the programme. General meetings, bulletins, and newsletters can be used as a means of promoting activities and keeping people informed. They can be supplemented by the activities of occupational health professionals and the person officially responsible for programme information. The most effective means is to confront people face-to-face. It is also important to include information on the local public organisations, sports clubs and private services offering various types of physical activity. Nowadays the internet is a helpful source.

Knowledgeable Experts

Motivating adults to change their life-style requires special knowledge about the activating process on the part of the participating experts. When groups of clients are comprised of sedentary or almost sedentary adults or elderly persons whose skill and fitness suffice only for simple physical activity programmes, making the programme interesting and meaningful demands completely different expertise from what traditional instructors' and teachers' education provides. The elderly population is a significant challenge both for professional physical activity instructors and for the schools which teach the instructors. The following list contains seven aids that help a person change his or her life-style and that should be taken into consideration when a physical activity programme is planned and carried out (Liikunta työkyvyn tukena, 1995; Sannamo, 1996; KKI-ohelma, 1998).

1) *Clear decision for change, which the person himself or herself makes.* The decision can be supported by or helped by an occupational health physician, an occupational health nurse or physiotherapist, and it can be facilitated by general information on the possibilities and significance of physical activity for the individual.

2) *Possibilities for physical activity in the everyday life of a person and knowledge about these possibilities.*

3) *Realistic objectives.* Setting a realistic objective requires input from physicians, physiotherapists, and instructors. Knowledge about the forms of physical activity used earlier, the fitness of the person, his or her functional capacity, and his or her areas of interest help in the search for the proper objectives.

4) *Periodic feedback and time restrictions.* A change in life-style has a better chance of succeeding if the objectives are linked to specific periods: weeks, months, and years. In the beginning it is important that progress be followed and that the workers receive feedback at short intervals. Positive results, and especially the fact that someone is following the progress, helps motivate a beginner. Later the interval between the objective, feedback and follow-up periods can be lengthened. Feedback and personal guidance and counselling from

experts are considered especially important. Face-to-face communication is significantly more effective than general comments, especially when personal characteristics and skill are in question. Positive family attitudes also help a worker make successful changes in life-style.

5) *Defeat of obstacles.* Regular activity for the elderly requires that the person overcome the obstacles to physical activity in daily life. The commonest reasons given are lack of time, tiredness, lack of companion or skill, lack of interest or facilities, health factors, lack of equipment or tools, cost, laziness and inability to get things done, housework, child care, and the like. Strategies to overcome these obstacles should be developed by the individual or the group in co-operation with the person responsible for the physical activity programme.

6) *Support and encouragement.* Encouragement to continue with the change can come from different sources and in many different forms: management, immediate supervisor, occupational health professional or colleagues. A personal reward that indicates that the employer has observed some change and wants to encourage the person to continue can be effective. Suitable rewards are different bonuses, which can be in the form of time, money, material, or public or other recognition.

7) *Stimulating experiences.* Changes in life-style are always associated with emotions. Positive experiences based on the joy, refreshment, relaxation, company, friends, instruction and possibilities to practice one's own sport are essential to the desire to continue being physically active. Women often emphasise the aesthetic experiences provided by physical activity or its possibilities for self-expression. For men the possibilities to compete and win, the exultation brought on by the effort and the excitement are important. It also helps if the activity is voluntary rather than forced.

Follow-up, Measurement and Tests as a Part of the Physical Activity Programme

The method used to follow the results of an enterprise's physical activity programme is chosen according to the goals set. Changes in the number of regularly physically active workers or changes in the mode of activity can be followed easily with the aid of a questionnaire and fitness card. If the objectives have been linked to functional capacity and work ability, tests that measure these characteristics should be used. Changes in the ability to cope, the work atmosphere and satisfaction with the physical activity programme can be followed best with different questionnaires. If the objectives are clear numerical or percentage changes in sickness absence, work productivity or premature retirement, calculation of the figures depicts the success of the programme. Part of the aforementioned means of follow-up can be done within the enterprise, but demanding fitness, functional capacity and work ability tests and calculations of productivity need the help of the experts who have become partners in the project.

In assessing the need for tests and measures it is best first to consider how they promote the primary objective of the programme: more and more regularly active workers. People can also be motivated to be physically active by means other than tests. In this manner more resources are available for putting the activity into effect. Excessive testing can also scare away the most important target group, the physically passive workers.

Measures directed towards fitness and participation in hobbies do have some advantages; for example, they make the initial planning easier and later provide feedback that lays a basis for developing the programme into a continual process. Data on the worker's initial condition - fitness or functional capacity - provide good indicators of the need for action. In this manner the services offered can be better specified and they can be tailored to meet the individual needs of the risk groups. Good results motivate both employees and employers, whereas poorer results than expected provide a reason for re-evaluating the activities.

Physical fitness and the amount of physical activity can be measured in many ways. One simple test is a self-assessment of the factors comprising fitness. A medical examination and discussion with a physician are applicable to determine the possible risks related to beginning a physically active life-style. Another good starting point for those who plan the programme is a questionnaire directed towards the work community as a whole; the questionnaire should also inquire about current daily activities and the worker's perception of his or her physical condition and ability to cope.

A good, simple and cheap means of following physical activity is a training log or fitness card. The log or card makes it possible to follow the regularity of the activity, its frequency, its contents and also its intensity, and it acts as a personal form of motivation and is a suitable aid for different forms of follow-up done at the workplace, for instance, the follow-up of physical activity participation, different competitions and rewards.

For larger groups simple group tests or a test battery are suitable. One such test battery, which includes body mass index, a walking test and body strength and flexibility can be found in the KKI programme published in *Työkunto nousuun* [Fitness to Work on the Rise], page 28-30. Many parties have developed computer-based group tests that, in addition to fitness results, give recommendations for continued training on the basis of the results. Currently, the most common such test in use is the UKK Walk Test.

The Finnish Institute of Occupational Health has developed a method suitable for the working environment. It is a computer-based *work* fitness profile for personal feedback, and it is meant to activate workers to follow their fitness level and be physically active on a regular basis. The profile is suitable for both management and workers. It includes measurements of musculoskeletal and aerobic fitness, the test instructions needed for the measurements, the work ability index and a questionnaire on life-style.

Heinola Model for a Successful Physical Education Project

One successful example of cooperation in executing a physical activity programme is the KKI model set up by the city of Heinola, which has a population of 30 000. The following organisations have participated in the planning and execution of the programme: the municipal recreational and sports bureau, occupational health care units and 30 small or middle-sized enterprises. The recreation and sports office was responsible for carrying out the programme. It marketed services to the enterprises, trained occupational health nurses and representatives of the enterprises and produced the needed services in conjunction with local sports clubs. Thirty enterprises, which employ a total of about 4000 persons, are participating in the programme. They have 30 different services or types of activity available weekly and complete freedom with respect to choice and frequency of participation. The services are very inexpensive for the enterprises. They pay

700-7000 Finnish marks per season (autumn/winter) depending on the number of employees. For this price all the services are freely available to all employees of all of the enterprises. The organisation, activity programme and management of the project are the responsibility of the project's secretary and an apprentice, both of whom were hired especially for the project. The physical activity groups are run by 10 trained instructors. The sessions are held outside work time. Occupational health care professionals are responsible for testing the fitness of the workers and motivating them to participate in the programme. The worker representatives keep their fellow workers informed and work to motivate them. Since the city of Heinola has donated the use of its facilities to this project, the costs are covered. About 1500 workers are regularly active within the scope of this project. The most popular forms of activity have been dancing, aerobics, belly dancing, water aerobics, and fitness training. Special services are offered to people with weight problems or people with illness symptoms. The model is very economic for both the worker and the city, and, at the same time, it is highly motivating for the workers. It offers versatile alternatives of physical activity and expert guidance.

References

Anttila, R. (1999). Kunnossa kaiken ikää –ohjelman arviointi. Liikunnan ja kansanterveyden julkaisuja 119. Jyväskylä: LIKES-tutkimuskeskus.

Anttila, R., Mertaniemi, M. (1997). Ehjä palveluketju tukee elämänmuutosta. Kipinät 1-2, 8. Kunnossa kaiken ikää –ohjelma.

Anttila, R., Mertaniemi, M. (1997). Miten ihmisen käyttäytyminen muuttuu. Kipinät 1-2/1997, s. 4-5. Helsinki: Kunnosa kaiken ikää – ohjelma.

Ahonen, G. (1995). Työkykyä ylläpitävän toiminnan taloudellinen merkitys. In E. Matikainen ja T. Aro (toim.), Hyvä työkyky (s. 25-30). Helsinki: Työterveyslaitos ja Eläkevakuutusosakeyhtiö Ilmarinen.

Baltes, P.B., Smith J. (1990). Toward a psychology of wisdom. In R.J. Sternberg (Ed.), Wisdom: Its nature, origins, and development (pp. 87-120). New York: Cambridge University Press.

Bergström, M., Huuskonen M., Koskinen K. (toim.) (1997). Työkyky yksilön, pienyrityksen ja yhteiskunnan menestystekijänä. Työ ja ihminen tutkimusraportti 10. Helsinki.

European Commission (1999). A Pan-EU Survey 1999. Brussels.

Ilmarinen J., Tuomi K., Klockars M. (1995). Ikääntyminen ja työkykyindeksin muutokset. Työ ja ihminen, tutkimusraportti 2. Työterveyslaitos. Helsinki.

Ilmarinen, J. (1995). Mikä suomalaisessa työssä ja elintavoissa luo työkykyä? In: J. Ilmarinen ja A. Järvikoski (toim.) Työkyky ja kuntoutus – nykytila ja tulevaisuus (s. 45-54) Helsinki: Työterveyslaitos ja Kuntoutussäätiö.

Ilmarinen, J. (1995). Työkykyä edistävät ja heikentävät tekijät. In: E. Matikainen ja T. Aro (toim.) Hyvä työkyky (s. 31-46). Helsinki: Työterveyslaitos ja Eläkevakuutusosakeyhtiö Ilmarinen.

Ilmarinen, J. (Ed.) (1991). The aging worker. *Scandinavian Journal of Work, Environment and Health*, 17, Suppl.1.

Ilmarinen, M. (1998). Henkilöstön työkyvyn tukeminen edistämällä fyysistä kuntoa. In: T. Aro ja E. Matikainen (toim.) *Työkyky hallintaan.* Helsinki: Työterveyslaitos ja Eläkevakuutusyhtiö Ilmarinen.

Ilmarinen, M. (toim.) (1993). *Liikunta lisää voimavaroja.* Liikunnan ja kansanterveyden julkaisuja 84. Helsinki.

Ilmarinen, M. (Ed.) (1993). Stronger through physical activity and sport. *Reports of physical culture and health*, no 87. Helsinki.

Kujala, A. (1995). Keski-ikäiset vieroksuvat ylipirteää superohjaajaa. *Liikunta ja tiede*, 32 (1) 51-53.

Kukkonen, R. ja Louhevaara, V. (1995). *Opas työolojen ja kunnon arvioimiseen ja kehittämiseen.* Työ ja liikunta 7. Helsinki: Työterveyslaitos.

Kunnon projekti Kuopiossa. (1993). Työturvallisuuskeskus, Työsuojelurahasto ja Kuopion kaupunki. Painatuskeskus.

Kyrklund, M. (2000). *Fysiokimppa - peruskurssi.* Vantaa: Fysiokimppa Oy.

Laakso, L., Telama, R., Vuolle, P. (1986). *Näin suomalaiset liikkuvat.* Jyväskylä: Likes-julkaisuja 50.

Louhevaara, V. ja Smolander, J. (1995). *Työkunto nousuun.* Helsinki: KKI-ohjelma ja Työterveyslaitos.

Mertaniemi M. ja Miettinen M. (1998) *Suuntana hyvinvointi – mitkä ovat liikunnan mahdollisuudet?* Liikunnan ja kansanterveyden julkaisuja 113. Jyväskylä.

Metteri, A. (1996) Näin projekti onnistuu. Esitelmä Terveysliikuntapäivillä 9-10.9.1996. Tampere: UKK-Instituutti.

Ruoppila, I. (1996). Elämänkaaren kehityspsykologia. In: E. Kiuru, (toim.), *Promootiokutsu* 17.5.1996. Jyväskylä: Jyväskylän yliopisto.

Ruoppila, I. (1996). Henkinen toiminakyky ja oppiminen. In: *Ikääntyvät työelämässä*. *Ikääntyvien työllistymisedellytysten parantamista selvittäneen komitean mietintö* (s. 193-212). Liiteosa. Komiteanmietintö 1996:14, Työministeriö, Helsinki.

Ruoppila, I., Suutama, T. (1994). Psyykkisen toimintakyvyn muutokset vanhetessa. In: J. Kuusinen ym. (toim) *Ikääntyminen ja työ* (s. 58-75). Helsinki: WSOY ja Työterveyslaitos.

Sannamo, M. (1994). Muutos yksilön elämäntavoissa. Asiantuntijaluento KKI-seminaarissa Haikossa 1.4.1994. Helsinki: Kunnossa kaiken ikää – ohjelma.

Shephard, R.J. (1990). The costs and benefits of exercise: an industrial perspective. In: *Fitness for the aged, disabled, and industrial worker. International Series on Sport Sciences*, 20, 189-204.

Vuori, I. (1996). *Tehokas, turvallinen terveysliikunta*. Helsinki: UKK-instituutti, Kunnossa kaiken ikää -ohjelma ja Kansaneläkelaitos.

English Non-Specialist Bibliography

Alvestad, B., Jensen, H.N., Larun, L., Palner, J., Rosberg, A., Saetre, U. (1998). Does physical exercise at the workplace have any effect on sick leave? *Tidsskr-Nor-Laegeforen*, 30 (11), 1718-1721.

Ashenden, R., Silagy, C., Weller, D. (1997). A systematic review of the effectiveness of promoting lifestyle change in general practice. *Family Practice*, 14 (2), 160-175.

Baltes, P.B., Smith, J. (1990). Toward a psychology of wisdom. In: Sternberg, R.J. (Ed.). *Wisdom: Its nature, origins, and development*. New York: Cambridge University Press, 87-120.

Bauer, R., Heller, R. (1985). United prevention project: 12-year follow-up of risk factors. *American Journal of Epidemiology,* 121 (4), 563-569.

Blue, C., Conrad, K. (1995). Adherence to worksite exercise programs: an integrative review of recent research. *AAOHN Journal (Official Journal of the American Association of Occupational Health Nurses),* 43 (2), 76-86.

Dishman, R.K., Oldenburg, B., Hearther, O., Shephard, R.J. (1998). Worksite physical activity interventions. *American Journal of Preventative Medicine,* 15 (4), 344-361.

Harland, J, White, M., Drinkwater, C., Chinn, D., Farr, L., Howel, D. (1999). The newcastle exercise project: a randomised controlled trial of methods to promote physical activity in primary care, *British Medical Journal,* 319, 828-832.

Heiric, M., Foote, A., Erfurt, J., Konopka, B. (1993). Work-site physical fitness programs. Comparing the impact of different program designs on cardiovascular risks. *Journal of Occupational Medicine,* 35 (5), 510-517.

Hillsdon, M., Thorogood, M., Amstoss, T., Morris, J. (1995). Randomised controlled trials of physical activity promotion in free living populations: a review. *Journal of Epidemiology and Community Health,* 49, 448-453.

Kriska, A., Bayles, C., Cauley, J., laporte, R., Sandler, R., Pambianco, G. (1986). A randomized exercise trial in older women: increase activity over two years and the factors associated with compliance. *Medicine and Science in Sports and Exercise,* 18 (5), 557-562.

Lombard, D., Lombard, T., Winett, R. (1995). Walking to meet health guidelines: The effect of prompting frequency and prompt structure. *Health Psychology,* 144 (2), 164-170.

Lovibond, S., Birrell, P., Langeluddecke, P. (1986). Changing coronary heart disease risk-factor status: the effects of three behavioral programs. *Journal of Behavioural Medicine,* 9 (5), 415-437.

Lusk, S.L. (1997). Health promotion and disease prevention in the worksite. School of Nursing, University of Michigan, USA. *Annual Review of Nursing Research*, 15, 187-213.

Marcus, B., Simkin-Silverman, L., Linnan, L., Taylor, E., Bock, B., Roberts, M., Rossi, J., Abrahams, D. (1998a). Evaluation of motivationally tailored vs standard self-help physical activity interventions at workplace. *American Journal of Health Promotion*, 12 (4), 246-253.

Marcus, B., Bock, B., Pinto, B., Forsyth, L., Roberts, M., Traficante, R. (1998b). Efficacy of an individualized, motivationally-tailored physical activity intervention. *Annals of Behavioural Medicine*, 20 (3), 174-180.

Olden, G., Crouse, S., Reynolds, C. (1989). Worker productivity, job satisfaction, and work related stress; the influence of an employee fitness program. *Fitness in business*, 198- 204.

Oja, P., Vuori, I., Paronen, O. (1998). Daily walking and cycling to work: their utility as health-enhancing physical activity. *Patient Education and Counselling*, 33, 87-94.

Ostwald, S. (1989). Changing employees´ dietary and exercise practices: an experimental study in a small company. *Journal of Occupational Medicine*, 31 (2), 90-96.

Peterson, T., Aldana, S. (1999). Improving exercise behaviour: an application of the stages of change model in a worksite setting. *American Journal of Health Promotion*, 13 (4), 229-232.

Prochaska, J., DiClemente, C. (1983). Stages and processes of self change in smoking: towards an integrative model of change. *Journal of Consultative Clinical Psychology*, 51, 390-395.

Reid, E.L., Morgan, R.W (1979). Exercise prescription: a clinical trial. *American Journal of Public Health*, 69 (6), 591-595.

Sallis, J.F., Bauman, A., Pratt, M. (1998). Environmental and policy interventions to promote physical activity. Department of Psychology, San

Diego State University, California 92120, USA. *American Journal of Preventative Medicine*, 15 (4), 379-397.

Sharpe, P., Connell, C. (1992). Exercise beliefs and behaviours among alder employees: a health promotion trial. *The Gerontological Society of America* 32 (4), 444-449.

Shephard, R.J. (1996). Worksite fitness and exercise programs; a review of methodology and health impact. *American Journal of Health Promotion.* 10 (6), 346-452.

Shephard, R.J. (1999). Do worksite exercise and health programs work. *The Physician and Sportsmedicine Online*, Feb 1999, 1-20.

Skargren, E., Öberg, B. (1998). Effects of an exercise programme on organisational, psychological, and physical work conditions, and psychosomatic symptoms. Scandinavian Journal of Rehabilitation Medicine, 30, 1-7.

Steptoe, A., Doherty, S., Rink, E., Kerry, S., Kendrick, T., Hilton, S. (1999). Behavioural counselling in general practice for the promotion of healthy behaviour among adults at increased risk of coronary heart disease: randomised trial. *British Medical Journal*, 319 (9), 943-947.

Tuomi, K., Ilmarinen, J, Seitsamo, J. et al. (1997). Summary of the Finnish research project (1981–1992) to promote the health and work ability of ageing workers. *Scandinavian Journal of Work and Environmental Health*, 23, Suppl 1, 66-71.

Wanzel, R. (1994). Decades of worksite fitness programmes. Progress or rhetoric? *Sports Medicine*, 17 (5), 324-337.

English Specialist Bibliography

Gomel, M., Oldenburg, B., Simpson, J., Owen, N. (1993). Work-site cardiovascular risk reduction: a randomized trial of health risk assessment, education, counselling, and incentives. *American Journal of Public Health*, 93 (9), 1231-1238.

Hillsdon, M., Thorogood, M. (1996). A systematic review of physical activity promotion strategies. *British Journal of Sports Medicine*, 30 (2), 84-89.

Ilmarinen, J. (Ed.). (1991). The aging worker. *Scandinavian Journal of Work and Environmental Health*, 17, Suppl.1.

Ilmarinen, J., Tuomi, K., Klockars, M. (1997). Changes in the work ability of active employees over an 11-year period. *Scandinavian Journal of Work and Environmental Health*, 23, Suppl 1, 49-57.

King, A., Haskel, I W., Taylor, B., Kraemer, H., DeBusk, R. (1991). Group-vs home-based exercise training in healthy older man and women. A community-based clinical trial. *Journal of the American Medical Association*, 266 (11), 1535-1542.

Kohl, H., Dunn, A., Marcus, B., Blair, S. (1998). A randomised trial of *Medicine and Science in Sports and Exercise*, 30 (2), 275-283.

Louhevaara, V. (1999). Physical exercise as a measure to maintain work ability. In: Ilmarinen J, Louhevaara V. (Eds.) *Finn-Age-Respect for the aging: Action programme to promote health, work ability and wellbeing of aging workers in 1990-1996. People and work research reports 26.* Finnish Institute of Occupational Health.

Shephard, R.J. (1990). The costs and benefits of exercise: an industrial perspective. In: *Fitness for the aged, disabled, and industrial worker. International Series on Sport Sciences*, 20, 189-204.

Suter, E., Martil, B. (1992). Predictors of exercise adoption and adherence of middle-aged sedentary men in a randomised controlled trial. *Clinical Journal of Sports Medicine*, 4, 261-267.

Assessing Physical Performance of Older Adults in a Community Setting

C. Jessie Jones and Roberta E. Rikli

Introduction

The rapid growth in the ageing population presents a number of health and economic challenges for individuals, families and governments throughout the world. In 1950, there were only 131 million people aged 65 and older; in 1994, that number had almost tripled to approximately 357 million world-wide. Between now and the year 2025, that number is expected to double again. According to the U.S. Bureau of Census (1996) projections, by the year 2020, between one-fifth and one-fourth of the population in the industrialised countries will be over the age of 65, and the fastest growing segment of that population will be persons aged 80 or older. As a result of the projected increased growth and longevity of the older population, identifying ways to promote *active* life expectancy, and reduce the number of years people live with chronic disabilities, has become a major challenge for gerontology researchers and practitioners throughout the world. Active life expectancy is defined as the number of expected years of physical, emotional, and intellectual vigour or functional well being (Katz, et al. 1983).

One of the most effective ways for reducing age-related decline leading to frailty is through early detection of physical weaknesses and proper adjustments in physical activity behaviours (Jackson, Beard, Wier, & Blair, 1995). It has been estimated that regular participation in moderate

Correspondence to: Prof. Dr. Roberta Rikli, Division of Kinesiology and Health Promotion, California State University, Fullerton, California, 92834 USA amounts of physical activity can effectively postpone physical disability for 10-20 years (American College of Sports Medicine, 1998; Astrand, 1992; Blair et al., 1989; Buchner & Wagner, 1992; Morey, Pieper, & Cornoni-Huntley, 1998; Paffenbarger et al., 1993). However, a limiting factor detecting physical weakness has been the lack of suitable performance measures that can identify the underlying physical parameters (i.e., strength, endurance, flexibility, and motor ability (i.e., power, agility, and dynamic balance) associated with physical impairments. Especially, there is a lack of valid "field-test" (non-laboratory) physical performance measures that can provide "continuous-scale" assessments across the wide spectrum of functional abilities among community residing older adults (Chandler & Hadley, 1996; Chodzko-Zajko, 1994; Rikli & Jones, 1997; Spirduso, 1995; Verbrugge & Jette, 1994).

Traditionally most physical performance tools have been developed to either assess the fitness level of younger people, or they have been designed to assess functional limitations of the more frail population (Buchner, Guralnik, & Cress, 1995; Rikli & Jones, 1997; Spirduso, 1995). The limitations of using the traditional fitness testing protocols designed for younger individuals (such as those involving treadmill, cycle ergometers, and strength equipment for 1RM testing) are that the test items generally are too difficult and/or unsafe for the majority of older adults; too time consuming and expensive, and often times require extensive training for test technicians. Therefore, such tests are not suitable for testing in community settings where most older adults reside.

On the other hand, tests designed to assess functional limitations in the more frail population are generally too easy for independently living older adults. The two most common scales used to measure functional limitations and the ability to live independently are Activities of Daily Living (ADL) and Instrumental Activities of Daily Living (IADL) (Katz, Ford, & Moskowitz, 1963; Lawton & Brody, 1969). ADLs include tasks such as bathing, eating, dressing, toileting, and getting in or out of a bed or chair. IADLs involve more complex physical and cognitive tasks such as handling personal finances, preparing meals, shopping, doing housework, walking, and travelling. A major limitation of these and numerous other instruments designed to measure functional limitations (outlined in reviews by Feinstein, Josephy, & Wells 1986; Spirduso, 1995; and Rikli & Jones, 1997) are they do not detect the gradual physiological declines that lead to the eventual loss of functional ability. As a result, physical decline is often not detected until late in the disability process.

In response to the need for improved assessment tools to measure the physiological status of older adults, a newly designed "functional fitness" test was developed and validated through research at the Lifespan Wellness Clinic at California State University, Fullerton (Rikli & Jones, 1999). The purpose of this paper is (1) to discuss the importance of assessing physical performance in older adults, (2) to describe Fullerton's new functional fitness test for older individuals, with appropriate translation from U.S. non-metric units to metric units, (3) to discuss guidelines for administering the tests in a community setting, and (4) to present performance norms found in the United States for each test item, again with appropriate translations into metric units.

Importance of Assessing Physical Performance in Older Adults

According to recently developed curriculum standards, individuals teaching physical activity/fitness programmes for older adults should have knowledge on selection, administration, and interpretation of appropriate health and activity screening and functional fitness assessments to provide a basis for designing appropriate activity programmes (Jones & Clark, 1998). Assessing the physical performance of older adults can help to (1) identify and predict people at risk of becoming functionally dependent, (2) provide meaningful individual feedback, (3) motivate people to set goals to improve scores, (4) plan more effective physical activity programmes, and (5) determine types of services or referrals required. Also, in an era of accountability for health care (Russek, Wooden, Ekedahl, & Bush, 1997), assessing physical performance can provide practitioners with excellent outcome data to document and justify the benefits of physical activity for older adults.

Traditionally, however, physical assessment has been lacking in many activity programmes for older adults. Common reasons stated for not including assessment are (1) lack of appropriate assessment tools for "independently living" older adults, (2) lack of training on how to conduct and interpret assessments, (3) lack of time and budget for assessments, (4) lack of enough space to conduct the testing, and (5) lack of performance standards to use for comparisons (Jones & Clark, 1998; Jones & Rikli, 1994; Schroeder, 1995). The Fullerton "functional fitness" test was specifically developed to be easy to administer and score, safe for older participants (from semi-frail to very active), and require minimal equipment, time and space.

The Fullerton Functional Fitness Test

The Fullerton Functional Fitness Test measures the physiological attributes which support behaviours needed to perform everyday activities required for independent living: aerobic capacity, flexibility, strength, motor agility/dynamic balance. Body mass index (BMI), an estimate of body composition was also included as a test item because of its relationship to disease and dysfunction (Shephard, 1997). Functional fitness, in relation to this test, is operationally defined as *having the physiological capacity to perform normal everyday activities safely and independently without undue fatigue.* The selection of test items was based on a number of criteria recommended by Rikli & Jones (1997), including that the test protocols (1) represent major functional fitness components, (2) meet acceptable scientific standards of test reliability and validity, (3) are capable of providing continuous-scale measurements across the wide range of ability levels typically found in the community-residing older adults, (4) reflect usual age-related changes in physical performance, (5) can detect physical changes due to age and/or physical activity participation, (6) are easy to administer and feasible for use in community settings, and (7) are able, in most cases, to be administered without physician approval.

Test Items
After over two years of refining the protocols to meet the established criteria above, seven test items (and one alternative) were selected to assess the major components of functional fitness. Reliability and validity information is presented in other resources (Jones & Rikli, 1999; Jones, Rikli, Max & Noffal, 1998; Rikli & Jones, 1999a; Rikli & Jones, 1999b). Also, a national advisory panel of noted researchers, programme leaders, and practitioners served as reviewers and consultants during the development of test materials and protocols. Descriptions of the test protocols are presented in Appendix A. Although the tests were developed using the common U.S.

non-metric measuring systems, we have added metric equivalents in parentheses.

Guidelines for Community Testing

Preliminary Information
The Fullerton Functional Fitness Test is designed to be easy to administer and feasible for use with independent older adults within the community setting. The test battery and its accompanying performance norms are especially useful to 1) identify areas of individual weakness to plan intervention programmes, 2) assess usual rates of change across age groups, 3) compare individual scores with others of the same gender and age group, 4) motivate older adults to set goals for improvement, and 4) to document programme effectiveness. The following are some guidelines which may assist practitioners in using this test battery in a community programme setting.

Ideally, people participating in testing should come to the facility and sign-up for a particular day and time for the assessments. At that time, each participant should be required to complete a background, medical and health questionnaire, an informed consent (information about the testing), and a medical clearance (if necessary). A medical clearance is recommended if (1) a physician has advised the person not to exercise because of a medical condition, (2) the person is currently experiencing chest pain, dizziness, or has exertional angina (chest tightness, pressure, pain, heaviness) during exercise, (3) the participant has experienced congestive heart failure, and/or (4) the person has uncontrolled high blood pressure (160/100 or above). Participants should also be directed at the time of signing to monitor their physical exertion level, to perform within their comfort zone (i.e., never to a point of over-exertion or beyond what they feel is safe), and to notify the leader if they feel any discomfort or experience any unusual symptoms. In addition, participants should be given written instructions to inform them to avoid heavy exertion and alcohol use for 24 hours prior to testing, to eat a light meal one hour prior to testing, to wear clothing and shoes appropriate for participating in physical activity, to bring a hat and sun glasses for walking outside, and to bring reading glasses, if necessary, for completing the score card. As a reminder to the participants, the assessment date and time can also be written on the top of the instructions.

Testing procedures

The tests can be administered either individually or in group settings. However, since testing is typically done in the community setting using small groups, the following scenario describes testing procedures for up to 24 participants per group. It is possible to test 24 people in a 60-90-minute time period using a "circuit" set-up within a large indoor area such as a community centre or gymnasium, and an indoor or outdoor area for the 6-min walk. In order to avoid a fatigue factor, the circuit stations should be arranged in the following order around the periphery of the room: (1) chair stand, (2) arm curl, (3) height and weight, (4) chair sit-and-reach, (5) up-and-go, and (6) back scratch. Equipment needed and complete test protocols, including scoring procedures, are given in Appendix A. We recommend utilising a trained group of older adult volunteers to administer the testing at each station. Generally, only one technician is needed for each station, except at the arm curl station where two technicians are needed. Volunteers can be trained with little effort.

On assessment day a physical activity instructor should lead the participants through an 8-10 minute general warm-up and flexibility routine. Just prior to testing, participants are instructed to *"do the best that they can, but to never push themselves to a point of over exertion or beyond what they think is safe for them"*. Following instructions, the participants are evenly divided and sent to one of the six stations to begin testing. The co-ordinator walks around the room to be sure the tests are being correctly administered. As testing is completed at each station, the groups rotate together in a clockwise order until all tests have been given. The 6-min walk test is administered as a group at the completion of all other tests. See instructions in Appendix A.

When it is not possible or convenient to administer the 6-min walk because of insufficient space or bad weather, the 2-min step test can be substituted as a measure of aerobic endurance. In this case the 2-min step is included with the height and weight station as part of the circuit, and an extra technician is assigned to station 3. See Appendix A for complete instructions on how to administer all tests. All test procedures have been previously pilot-tested and found to produce reliable scores (Jones & Rikli, 1999; Jones, Rikli, Max & Noffal, 1998; Rikli & Jones, 1998; Rikli & Jones, 1999a).

Performance Norms for Test Items

A study in the United States was conducted to develop national normative scores for the tests. The study population consisted of 7,183 participants (aged 60-94 years) from 267 sites in 21 different states (Rikli & Jones, 1999b). The results include 5-year age group norms for each test item for both men and women (refer to Appendix B). Findings indicated that across all variables and most age groups, there was a consistent pattern of decline in performance from age 60-94. The amount of decline typically was in the 30-40 % range across the 3.5 decades, resulting in an approximate 1 % per year, or 10 % per decade loss in strength, endurance, and agility/balance scores. Also, there were significant gender differences on all test items. Women scored significantly better than men on the lower and upper body flexibility tests, and men scored significantly better than women on the lower and upper body strength tests, aerobic endurance, and agility/dynamic balance (Rikli & Jones, 1999b).

In summary, according to test administrators who assisted with the national study, the Fullerton Functional Fitness Test for Older Adults was easy to administer and score, fun and safe for the participants, and very valuable for programme planning and evaluation. In addition, we believe the test battery meets the standards of scientific rigor, and the test items can measure a wide-range of physical abilities typically found among older adults in a community setting. Most importantly, this test battery can help to identify areas of weakness before functional limitations develop so that proper interventions can be implemented to prevent or postpone the onset of physical disability among older adults.

We encourage other countries to use these tests to assess their populations so that international comparisons can be made relative to functional ageing across cultures. It would be critical, however, that all established methods and procedures be strictly followed if meaningful comparisons are going to be made across groups. Also, it would be important that similar populations be assessed. The criteria for inclusion in the U.S. normative study were that participants be independently living within the community and ambulatory without the use of assistive devices.

References

American College of Sports Medicine. (1998). Position stand: Exercise and physical activity for older adults. *Medicine and Science in Sport and Exercise*, 30, 992-1008.

Astrand, P. (1992). Why exercise? *Medicine and Science in Sports and Exercise*, 24, 153-162.

Blair, S. N., Kohl, H.W., Paffenbarger, R.S., Clark, D.G., Cooper, K.H., & Gibbons, L.W. (1989). Physical fitness and all-cause mortality: A prospective study of healthy men and women. *Journal of the American Medical Association*, 262, 2395-2401.

Buchner, D.M., & Wagner, E.H. (1992). Preventing frail health. *Health Promotion and Disease Prevention*, 8, 1-17.

Buchner, D.M., Guralnik, J.M., & Cress, M.E. (1995). The clinical assessment of gait, balance, and mobility in older adults. In L.Z. Rubenstein, D. Wieland, & R. Bernabei (Eds.), *Geriatric assessment technology: The state of the art* (pp. 75-89). Milano: Editrice Kurtis.

Chandler, J.M., & Hadley, E.C. (1996). Exercise to improve physiologic and functional performance in old age. *Clinics in Geriatric Medicine*, 12, 761-784.

Chodzko-Zajko, W. (1994). Assessing physical performance in older populations (Editorial). *Journal of Aging and Physical Activity*, 2, 103-104.

Feinstein, A.R., Josephy, B.R., & Wells, C.K. (1986). Scientific and clinical problems in indexes of functional disability. *Annals of Internal Medicine*, 105, 413-420.

Jackson, A.S., Beard, E.F., Wier, L.T., Ross, R.M., Stuteville, J.E., & Blair, S.N. (1995). Changes in aerobic power of men, ages 25-70 years. *Medicine and Science in Sports and Exercise*, 27, 113-120.

Jones, C.J. & Clark, J. (1998). National standards for preparing senior fitness instructors. *Journal of Aging and Physical Activity*, 6, 207-221.

Jones, C.J., & Rikli, R.E. (1999). A 30-second chair stand test as a measure of lower body strength in older adults. *Research Quarterly for Exercise and Sport, 70*, 113-119.

Jones, C.J. & Rikli, R.E. (1994). A revolution in aging: Implications for curriculum development and professional preparation in physical education. *Journal of Aging and Physical Activity, 2*, 261-272.

Jones, C.J., Rikli, R.E., Max, J., & Guillermo, G. (1998). The reliability and validity of a chair sit-and-reach test as a measure of hamstring flexibility in older adults. *Research Quarterly for Exercise and Sport, 69*, 338-343.

Katz, S., Ford, A.B., & Moskowitz, R.W. (1963). Studies of illness in the aged - The index of ASL: A standardized measure of biological and psychosocial function. *Journal of the American Medical Association, 185*, 914-918.

Katz, S. et al. (November 17, 1983). Active life expectancy. *The New England Journal of Medicine*, 1218-1224.

Lawton, M.P., & Brody, E.M. (1969). Assessment of older people: Self-maintaining and instrumental activities of daily living. *Gerontologist, 9*, 179-186.

Morey, M.C., Pieper, C.F., & Cornoni-Huntley, J. (1998). Physical fitness and functional limitations in community-dwelling older adults. *Medicine and Science in Sports and Exercise, 30*, 715-723.

Rikli, R.E., & Jones, C.J. (1999a). The development and validation of a functional fitness test for community-residing older adults. *Journal of Aging and Physical Activity, 7*, 129-161.

Rikli, R.E., & Jones, C. J. (1999b). Functional fitness normative scores for community-residing older adults, ages 60-94. *Journal of Aging and Physical Activity, 7*, 162-181.

Rikli, R.E., & Jones, C.J. (1998). The reliability and validity of a 6-minute walk test as a measure of physical endurance in older adults. *Journal of Aging and Physical Activity, 6*, 363-375.

Rikli, R.E., & Jones, C.J. (1997). Assessing physical performance in independent older adults: Issues and guidelines. *Journal of Aging and Physical Activity*, 5, 244-261.

Russek, L., Wooden, M., Ekedahl, S., & Bush, A. (1997). Attitudes toward standardized data collection. *Physical Therapy*, 77, 714-729.

Schroeder, J. (1995). A comprehensive survey of older adult exercise programs in two California communities. *Journal of Aging and Physical Activity* 3, 290-298.

Shephard, R.J. (1997). *Aging, physical activity, and health*. Champaign, IL: Human Kinetics.

Spirduso, W.W. (1995). *Physical Dimensions of Aging*. Champaign, IL: Human Kinetics.

U.S. Bureau of the Census. (1996). *Sixty-five plus in the United States: Current population reports* (P23-190). Washington, DC: U.S. Department of Commerce.

Verbrugge, L. M & Jette, A. M. (1994). The disablement process. *Social Science and Medicine*, 38, 1-14.

Additional Readings for Non-Specialists

American College of Sports Medicine. (1998). *ACSM fitness book.* Champaign: Human Kinetics.

American College of Sports Medicine. (1997). *ACSM's Exercise management for persons with chronic diseases and disabilities*. Champaign, IL: Human Kinetics.

American Council on Exercise. (1998). *Exercise for older adults: ACE's guide for fitness professionals*. Champaign, IL: Human Kinetics.

Clark, J. (1992). Full life fitness: A complete exercise program for mature adults. Champaign: Human Kinetics.

Ettinger, W.H., Mitchell, B.S., & Blair, S.N. (1996). *Fitness after 50*. St Louis: Beverly Cracom Publications.

Harris, S., & Hurley, O. (1995). *Who? Me? Exercise? Safe exercise for people over 50*. Reston, VA: AAHPERD Publications.

Lamb, D.R., Gisolfi, C.V., & Nadel, E. (1995). *Perspectives in exercise science and sports medicine.* Carmel, IN: Cooper Publishing Group.

Nelson, M. & Wernick, S. (1998). *Strong women stay slim*. New York: Bantam Books.

Nelson, M. & Wernick, S. (1986). *Strong women stay young*. New York: Bantam Books.

Newman, L.A. (1995). *Maintaining function in older adults*. Boston: Butterworth-Heinemann.

Osness, W. (1998). *Exercise and the older adults*. Reston, VA: AAHPERD Publications.

Rowe, J.W., & Kahn, R.L. (1998). *Successful aging*. New York: Pantheon.

Shephard, R.J. (1997). *Aging, physical activity, and health*. Champaign: Human Kinetics.

Van Norman, K.A. (1995). *Exercise programming for older adults*. Champaign: Human Kinetics.

Westcott, W.L. (1998). *Strength training past 50*. Champaign: Human Kinetics.

Authors' Notes

This work was supported by PacifiCare/Secure Horizons.

Appendix A: Functional Fitness Test For Older Adults

The following are specific directions for administering each of the test items. To assure scoring accuracy and interpretation, strict adherence to all test instructions is essential. Throughout all testing, participants should be instructed to *"do the best they can on the tests, but to never push themselves to a point of over exertion or beyond what they think is safe for them."* Prior to testing, people need to participate in a 5-10 minute warm-up and general stretch routine.

Based on guidelines established by the American College of Sports Medicine (1995) and on input from our medical consultants, these tests are safe for the majority of community-residing older adults without medical screening, and pose risks similar to engaging in moderate physical activity. Persons who *should not* take the tests without physician approval are those who:

- have been advised by their doctors not to exercise because of a medical condition,
- are currently experiencing chest pain, dizziness, or have exertional angina (chest tightness, pressure, pain, heaviness) during exercise,
- have experienced congestive heart failure, and/or
- have uncontrolled high blood pressure (greater than 160/100).

30-Second Chair Stand	
Purpose	To assess lower body strength.
Equipment	Stopwatch, straight back or folding chair (without arms) seat height approximately 17" (43.18 cm). For safety purposes, the chair should be placed against a wall, or in some other way stabilised, to prevent it from moving during the test.
Protocol	The test begins with the participant seated in the middle of the chair, back straight, and feet flat on the floor. Arms are crossed at the wrists and held against the chest. On the signal "go" the participant rises to a *full stand* and returns back to a fully seated position. The participant is encouraged to complete as many full stands as possible within a 30-second time limit. Following a demonstration by the tester, a practice trial of one or two repetitions should be given to check for proper form, followed by one 30 second test trial.
Scoring	The score is the total number of stands executed correctly within 30-seconds. If the participant is more than half way up at the end of 30-seconds, it counts as a full stand.

Arm Curl	
Purpose	To assess upper body strength.
Equipment	Wrist watch with second hand, straight back or folding chair (without arms) seat height approximately 17" (43.18 cm), hand weights - dumbbells - 5 lbs. (2.27 kg.) for women and 8 lbs. (3.63 kg) for men.
Protocol	The participant is seated on a chair, back straight and feet flat on the floor, and with the dominant side of the body close to the edge. The weight is held at the side in the dominant hand (handshake grip). The test begins with the arm in the down position beside the chair, perpendicular to the floor. At the signal "go" the participant turns the palm up while curling the arm through a full range of motion, and then returns to the fully extended position. At the down position the weight should have returned to the handshake grip position.
	The examiner kneels (or sits in a chair) next to the participant on the dominant arm side, placing his/her fingers on the person's mid-bicep to stabilise the upper arm from moving, and to assure that a full curl is made (participant's forearm should squeeze examiner's fingers). It is important that the participant's upper arm remains stabilised (still) throughout the test.
	The examiner may also need to position his/her other hand behind the elbow so that the person will know when full extension has been reached, and to prevent a "back swinging motion" of the arm.
	The participant is encouraged to execute as many curls as possible within the 30-second time limit. Following a demonstration by the examiner, a practice trial of one or two repetitions should be given to check for proper form, followed by one 30-second trial.
Scoring	The score is the total number of curls made correctly within 30 seconds. If the arm is more than half way up at the end of the 30-seconds, it counts as a curl.

6-Minute Walk Test	
Purpose	To assess aerobic endurance.
Equipment	Stopwatch, long measuring tape, cones, Popsicle sticks, chalk, masking tape (or some other type of marker). For safety purposes, chairs should be positioned at several points along the outside of the walkway.
Set-up	The test involves assessing the maximum distance that can be walked in 6 minutes along a 50-yard (45.72 meter) course, marked into 5-yard (4.57 meter) segments. Participants continuously walk around a measured lap throughout the 6-minute period, trying to cover as much distance as possible. The inside perimeter of the measured distance should be marked with cones and the 5-yard (4.57 meter) segments with masking tape or chalk. The walking area should be well lit, with the surface non -slippery and level.
Protocol	To keep track of distance walked, a Popsicle stick (or similar object) can be given to the participant each time he/she rounds a cone, or partners

	can mark on a score card each time a lap is completed. Two or more participants should be tested at a time, with starting times staggered (10 seconds apart) so that participants do not walk in clusters or pairs. When testing several people at a time, numbers should be placed on the participants to indicate the order of starting and stopping (nametags can be placed on their shirts). On the signal "go", participants are instructed to walk as fast as possible (not run) around the course as many times as they can within the time limit. If necessary, participants may stop and rest (sit on chairs provided), then resume walking. The timer should move to the inside of the marked area after everyone has started. To assist with pacing, elapsed time should be "called out" when participants are approximately half done, when 2 minutes are left, and when 1 minute is left. At the end of 6 minutes, participants (at 10-sec intervals) are instructed to "stop" and move to the right, where an assistant will record the score. To assist with proper pacing and to improve scoring accuracy, a practice test should be given prior to the test day.
Safety	The test should be discontinued if at any time participants shows signs of dizziness, pain, nausea, or undue fatigue. At the end of the test the participant should *slowly* walk around for about a minute to cool-down.
Scoring	The score is the total number of yards walked in 6 minutes to the nearest 5-yard (4.57 meter) indicator. The test administrator or aide records the nearest 5-yard (4.57 meter) mark.
Sample	50 (45.72 meter) yards measured into 5-yard (4.57 meter) segments.

2 Minute Step-in-Place	
Purpose	An alternative test to assess aerobic endurance.
Equipment	Stop watch, tape measure or 30-inch (76.2) piece of cord, masking tape, and a mechanical counter (if possible) to ensure accurate counting of steps.
Set-up	The proper (minimum) knee stepping height for each participant is at a level even with the mid-way point between the patella (middle of the knee cap) and the iliac crest (top hip bone). This point can be determined using a tape measure, or by simply stretching a piece of cord from the patella to the iliac crest, then doubling it over to determine the mid-way point. To monitor correct knee height when stepping, books can be stacked on an adjacent table, or a ruler can be attached to a chair or wall with masking tape marking the proper knee height.
Protocol	On the signal "go" the participant begins stepping (not running) in place, starting with the right leg, and continues as many steps as possible within the time period. Although both knees must be raised to the correct height to be counted, the tester only counts the number of times the right knee reaches the correct height. The counter also serves as a spotter in case of loss of balance and assures that the subject maintains proper knee height. As soon as proper knee height can not be maintained, the participant is asked to stop--or to stop and rest until proper form can be regained. Stepping may be resumed if the 2-minute time period has not elapsed. If necessary, one hand can be placed on the table or chair to assist in maintaining balance.

	To assist with proper pacing and to improve scoring accuracy, a practice test should be given prior to the test day. On test day, the examiner should demonstrate the procedure and allow the participants to practice briefly to recheck their understanding of the protocol.
Safety	At the end of the test the participant should slowly walk around for about a minute to cool-down.
Scoring	The score is the total number of times the *right knee* reaches the minimum height. To assist with pacing, subjects should be told when one minute has passed and when there are 30 seconds to go.

Chair Sit and Reach Test	
Purpose	To assess lower body (primarily hamstring) flexibility.
Equipment	Straight back or folding chair 17" (43.18 cm) (approx. seat height) and an approx. 18" (45.72 cm) ruler. For safety purposes, the chair should be placed against a wall and checked to see that it remains stable (doesn't tip forward) when the person sits on the front edge.
Protocol	Starting in a sitting position on a chair, the participant moves forward until she/he is sitting on the front edge of the chair. The crease between the top of the leg and the buttocks should be even with the edge of the chair seat. Keeping one leg bent and *foot flat on the floor*, the other leg (the preferred leg*) is extended straight in front of the hip, with heel on floor and foot flexed (at approx. 90°). With the extended leg as straight as possible (but not hyperextended), the participant slowly bends forward *at the hip joint* (spine should remain as straight as possible, with the head in line with spine, not tucked) sliding the hands (one on top of the other with the tips of the middle fingers even) down the extended leg in an attempt to touch the toes. The reach must be held for two seconds. If the extended knee starts to bend, ask the participant to slowly sit back until knee is straight before scoring. Participants should be reminded to exhale as they bend forward, avoid bouncing or rapid, forceful movements, and never stretch to the point of pain. Following a demonstration by the tester, the participant is asked to determine the preferred leg. The participant is then given two practice (stretching) trials on that leg, followed by two test trials.
Scoring	Using about an 18" (45.72 cm) ruler, the scorer records the number of inches a person is short of reaching the toe (minus score) or reaches beyond the toe (plus score). The middle of the toe at the end of the shoe represents a zero score. Record both test scores to the nearest 1/2 inch (cm), and circle the "best" score. The "best" score is used to evaluate performance. Be sure to indicate "minus" or "plus" on the score card.

*The preferred leg is defined as the one which results in the better score. Obviously, it is important to work on flexibility on both sides of the body, but for the sake of time, only the "better" side has been used in developing norms.

Back Scratch	
Purpose	To assess upper body (shoulder) flexibility.
Equipment	About an 18" (45.72 cm) ruler (half of a yardstick).
Protocol	In a standing position, the participant places the preferred hand* over the same shoulder, palm down and fingers extended, reaching down the middle of the back as far as possible (elbow pointed up). The hand of other arm is placed behind the back, palm up, reaching up as far as possible in an attempt to touch or overlap the extended middle fingers of both hands.
	Without moving the participant's hands, the tester helps to see that the middle fingers of each hand are directed toward each other. The participants are not allowed to grab their fingers together and pull.
	Following a demonstration by the tester, the participant is asked to determine the preferred hand. The participant is then given two practice (stretching) trials, followed by two test trials.
Scoring	The distance of overlap, or distance between the tips of the middle fingers is measured to the nearest 1/2 inch (cm). Minus scores (-) are given to represent the distance short of touching middle fingers; plus scores (+) represent the degree of overlap of middle fingers. Record both test scores and circle the "best" score. The "best" score is used to evaluate performance. Be sure to indicate minus or plus on the score card.

*The preferred hand is defined as the one which results in the better score. Although, it is important to work on flexibility on both sides of the body, only the "better" has been used in developing norms.

8' Up and Go	
Purpose	To assess physical mobility - involves power, speed, agility, and dynamic balance.
Equipment	Stop watch, tape measure, cone (or similar marker), and straight back or folding chair, approximate seat height approx. 17" (43.18 cm).
Set-up	The chair should be positioned against a wall or in some other way secured so that it does not move during the testing. The chair should also be in a clear, unobstructed area, facing a cone marker exactly 8 ft (243.84 cm) away (measured from a point on the floor even with the front edge of the chair to the back of the marker). There should be at least 4 feet (121.92 cm) of clearance beyond the cone to allow ample turning room for the participant.
Protocol	The test begins with the participant fully seated in the chair (erect posture), hands on thighs, and feet flat on the floor (one foot slightly in front of the other). On the signal "go" the person gets up from the chair (may push off thighs or chair), walks as quickly as possible around the cone (either side), and returns to the chair. The participant should be told that this is a "timed" test and that the object is to walk as quickly as possible (without running) around the cone and back to the chair. The tester should serve as a "spotter," standing midway between the chair and the cone, ready to assist the participant, in case of a loss of balance. For

	reliable scoring, the tester must start the timer on "go" whether or not the person has started to move, and "stop" the timer at the exact instant the person sits in the chair. Following a demonstration, the participant should walk through the test one time as a practice, and then is given two test trials. Participants should be reminded that the time does not stop until they are fully seated in the chair.
Scoring	The score is the time elapsed from the signal "go" until the subject returns to a seated position on the chair. Record both test scores to the nearest $1/10^{th}$ second and circle the "best" score (lowest time). The "best" score is used to evaluate performance.

Appendix B

Table 1. Age-group percentiles: Women

Chair Stand	60-64	65-69	70-74	75-79	80-84	85-89	90-94
(# of stands)	(n=595)	(n=1,027)	(n=1,240)	(n=937)	(n=502)	(n=305)	(n=141)
%ile Rank							
10th	9	9	8	7	6	5	2
25th	12	11	10	10	9	8	4
50th	15	14	13	12	11	10	8
75th	17	16	15	15	14	13	11
90th	20	18	18	17	16	15	14

Arm Curl	60-64	65-69	70-74	75-79	80-84	85-89	90-94
(# of curls)	(n=598)	(n=1,034)	(n=1,258)	(n=953)	(n=519)	(n=329)	(n=146)
%ile Rank							
10th	10	10	9	8	8	7	6
25th	13	12	12	11	10	10	8
50th	16	15	15	14	13	12	11
75th	19	18	17	17	16	15	13
90th	22	21	20	20	18	17	16

6 min Walk	60-64	65-69	70-74	75-79	80-84	85-89	90-94
(#meters walked	(n=356)	(n=617)	(n=728)	(n=513)	(n=276)	(n=152)	(n=79)
%ile Rank							
10th	453	402	384	334	283	238	178
25th	498	457	439	393	352	311	251
50th	553	521	503	466	421	389	320
75th	604	581	562	535	494	466	402
90th	649	636	617	599	558	544	476

2 min Step	60-64	65-69	70-74	75-79	80-84	85-89	90-94
(# of full steps)	(n=264)	(n=491)	(n=597)	(n=489)	(n=279)	(n=167)	(n=61)
%ile Rank							
10th	60	57	53	52	46	42	31
25th	75	73	68	68	60	55	44
50th	91	90	84	84	75	70	58
75th	107	107	101	100	91	85	72
90th	122	123	116	115	104	98	85

Chair Sit & Reach	60-64	65-69	70-74	75-79	80-84	85-89	90-94
(# of cm from toes	(n=591)	(n=1037)	(n=1250)	(n=954)	(n=514)	(n=332)	(n=151)
%ile Rank							
10th	-8	-8	-9	-10	-11	-11	-18
25th	-1	-1	-3	-4	-5	-6	-11
50th	5	5	4	3	1	-1	-5
75th	13	11	10	9	8	6	3
90th	18	17	15	14	13	11	9

Back Scratch	60-64	65-69	70-74	75-79	80-84	85-89	90-94
(cm between finger	(n=592)	(n=1030)	(n=1246)	(n=946)	(n=517)	(n=323)	(n=148)
%ile Rank							
10th	-14	-15	-17	-19	-20	-25	-29
25th	-8	-9	-10	-13	-14	-18	-20
50th	-1	-3	-4	-5	-6	-10	-11
75th	4	4	3	1	0	-3	-3
90th	10	9	8	8	6	5	5

8' Up and Go	60-64	65-69	70-74	75-79	80-84	85-89	90-94
(# of sec.)	(n=594)	(n=1033)	(n=1244)	(n=938)	(n=497)	(n=306)	(n=142)
%ile Rank							
10th	6.7	7.1	8.0	8.3	10.0	11.1	13.5
25th	6.0	6.4	7.1	7.4	8.7	9.6	11.5
50th	5.2	5.6	6.0	6.3	7.2	7.9	9.4
75th	4.4	4.8	4.9	5.2	5.7	6.2	7.3
90th	3.7	4.1	4.0	4.3	4.4	5.1	5.3

Body Mass Index	60-64	65-69	70-74	75-79	80-84	85-89	90-94
(kg/m^2)	(n=572)	(n=1016)	(n=1213)	(n=916)	(n=504)	(n=337)	(n=149)
%ile Rank							
10th	19.6	19.8	20.3	19.8	19.6	19.5	18.3
25th	22.8	23.0	23.1	22.5	22.0	21.8	21.1
50th	26.3	26.5	26.1	25.4	24.7	24.3	24.1
75th	29.8	30.0	29.1	28.3	27.4	26.8	27.1
90th	33.0	33.2	31.9	31.0	30.0	29.0	29.5

Table 2. Age-group percentiles: Men

Chair Stand	60-64	65-69	70-74	75-79	80-84	85-89	90-94
(# of stands)	(n=230)	(n=460)	(n=498)	(n=434)	(n=226)	(n=108)	(n=71)
%ile Rank							
10th	11	9	9	8	7	6	5
25th	14	12	12	11	10	8	7
50th	16	15	15	14	12	11	10
75th	19	18	17	17	15	14	12
90th	22	21	20	19	18	17	15

Arm Curl	60-64	65-69	70-74	75-79	80-84	85-89	90-94
(# of curls)	(n=229)	(n=458)	(n=498)	(n=440)	(n=232)	(n=113)	(n=71)
%ile Rank							
10th	13	12	11	10	10	8	7
25th	16	15	14	13	13	11	10
50th	19	18	17	16	16	14	12
75th	22	21	21	19	19	17	14
90th	25	25	24	22	21	19	17

6 min Walk	60-64	65-69	70-74	75-79	80-84	85-89	90-94
(#meters walked	(n=144)	(n=281)	(n=294)	(n=23)	(n=130)	(n=60)	(n=48)
%ile Rank							
10th	508	457	439	361	338	270	197
25th	578	512	498	430	407	348	279
50th	617	576	558	508	480	434	370
75th	672	640	622	585	553	521	457
90th	722	700	681	654	622	604	540

2 min Step	60-64	65-69	70-74	75-79	80-84	85-89	90-94
(# of full steps)	(n=92)	(n=211)	(n=225)	(n=226)	(n=119)	(n=50)	(n=38)
%ile Rank							
10th	74	72	66	56	56	44	36
25th	87	86	80	73	71	59	52
50th	101	101	95	91	87	75	69
75th	115	116	110	109	103	91	86
90th	128	130	125	125	118	106	102

Chair Sit & Reach	60-64	65-69	70-74	75-79	80-84	85-89	90-94
(# of cm from toes	(n=228)	(n=461)	(n=494)	(n=434)	(n=231)	(n=113)	(n=74)
%ile Rank							
10th	-15	-15	-17	-18	-20	-20	-23
25th	-6	-8	-9	-10	-14	-14	-17
50th	1	0	-1	-3	-5	-6	-9
75th	10	8	6	5	4	1	1
90th	17	15	14	13	11	8	5

Back Scratch	60-64	65-69	70-74	75-79	80-84	85-89	90-94
(cm between finger	(n=228)	(n=457)	(n=489)	(n=430)	(n=226)	(n=113)	(n=73)
%ile Rank							
10th	-25	-27	-28	-30	-32	-32	-34
25th	-17	-19	-20	-23	-24	-25	-27
50th	-9	-10	-11	-14	-14	-15	-18
75th	0	-3	-3	-5	-5	-8	-10
90th	6	5	5	3	3	0	-3

8' Up and Go	60-64	65-69	70-74	75-79	80-84	85-89	90-94
(# of sec.)	(n=229)	(n=461)	(n=492)	(n=436)	(n=227)	(n=106)	(n=72)
%ile Rank							
10th	6.4	6.5	6.8	8.3	8.7	10.5	11.8
25th	5.6	5.7	6.0	7.2	7.6	8.9.	10.0
50th	4.7	5.1	5.3	5.9	6.4	7.2	8.1
75th	3.8	4.3	4.2	4.6	5.2	5.3	6.2
90th	3.0	3.8	3.6	3.5	4.1	3.9	4.4

Body Mass Index	60-64	65-69	70-74	75-79	80-84	85-89	90-94
(kg/m^2)	(n=228)	(n=460)	(n=491)	(n=491)	(n=230)	(n=114)	(n=69)
%ile Rank							
10th	22.0	22.1	21.6	21.4	21.7	21.8	20.2
25th	24.6	24.7	24.0	23.8	23.8	23.3	22.4
50th	27.4	27.5	26.6	26.4	26.1	24.9	24.9
75th	30.2	30.3	29.2	29.0	28.4	26.5	27.4
90th	32.8	32.9	31.6	31.4	30.5	28.0	29.6

Resources and Contacts

1. INTERNATIONAL ORGANISATIONS

International Council of Sport Science and Physical Education (ICSSPE)

ICSSPE is an umbrella organisation with a diverse range of over 220 member organisations world-wide. The Council promotes and disseminates a wide range of scientific information, and has a co-ordinating function with national and international organisations, as well as a close relationship with UNESCO and the IOC. It also plays an active role in the Network on Active Living, initiated by the WHO, and supports programmes aimed at developing physical activity and health for all population groups.

A comprehensive website is updated on a regular basis to share knowledge, report events, and announce newly published resources. It is just one of the many ways used to build stronger international co-operation and bridge the gap between developed and developing countries. See the link to the SIRC Calendar for details about upcoming events.

ICSSPE/CIEPSS Executive Office	Tel:	+49 30 805 00360
Am Kleinen Wannsee 6	Fax:	+49 30 805 6386
14109 Berlin	E-mail:	icsspe@icsspe.org
GERMANY	Internet:	www.icsspe.org

International Society for Aging and Physical Activity (ISAPA)

An international not-for-profit society promoting research, clinical practice, and public policy initiatives in the area of aging and physical activity. ISAPA is divided into four major geographic regions, each represented by two board members with their own web page. Membership is open to professionals and students with an interest in gerontology, physical activity, exercise science, fitness, or other related fields.

An official *Journal of Aging and Physical Health*, Resource Center, Newsletter, Calendar of Events, and hundreds of physical activity and aging links are available on their website. Also see links to laboratories, universities, and other national and local sites, as well as information about courses in physical activity and aging. If you are searching for a particular testing protocol, wanting to advertise a forthcoming event, or simply if you want to comment on some aspect of activity and aging, feel free to use their bulletin board.

Prof. Dr. Wojtek Chodzko-Zajko, ISAPA President School of Exercise, Leisure and Sport Kent State University 163 MGA Kent, OH 44242 USA	Tel: Fax: E-mail: Internet:	+1 330 2837286 +1 330 6724106 isapa@kent.edu www.isapa.org

World Health Organization (WHO)
Ageing and Health Programme (AHE)

The ultimate objective of the WHO Ageing and Health Programme (AHE) is to establish a global strategy on healthy ageing by promoting health and well-being throughout the entire lifespan, as well as ensuring the availability and provision of comprehensive and holistic health care to elderly populations. In doing so, the programme has six integrated components: information strengthening; information dissemination; advocacy; informed research; training; and policy development.

AHE is planning the establishment of "global centres" on ageing and health with a particular focus on policy development for healthy ageing in developing countries. Its most precious resource is its continuously expanding network of individuals, academic institutes, non-governmental agencies and governmental offices. A comprehensive website provides links to an overview, brief history, scope of the challenge, global partnerships, information about World Health Day, and the Geneva International Network on Ageing (GINA).

Dr. Alexandre Kalache	Tel:	+41 22 7913404
WHO Ageing and Health	Fax:	+41 22 7914839
Avenue Appia 20	E-mail:	Kalachea@who.ch
CH-1211 Geneva 27	Internet:	www.who.int/ageing
SWITZERLAND		

World Heart Federation (WHF)

The World Heart Federation is composed of heart foundations from around the world with the purpose of raising funds to support research, professional and public education, and community programmes. Their scientific arm is composed of ten scientific councils carrying on multi-national research projects, teaching, training and treatment, as well as basic research, prevention and rehabilitation.

Dr. Tak-Fu TSE, President	Tel:	+852 2526 6081
World Heart Federation	Fax:	+852 2845 2513
16th floor, Central Building	E-mail:	drtftse@vitagreen.com
1-3 Pedder Street	Internet:	www.worldheart.org/
Central, Hong Kong		

European Network for the Promotion of Health-Enhancing Physical Activity

An initiative of the UKK Institute in Tampere Finland.

UKK Institute	Tel:	+358 32 829202
P.O. Box 30	Fax:	+358 32 829200
33501 Tampere	E-mail:	losapi@uta.fi
Finland		

Europe on the Move Information Network

NOC*NSF   Tel: +31 264 834 709
P.O. Box 302   Fax: +31 264 834 732
6800 AH Arnhem   E-mail:sport.gezondheid@noc-nsf.nl
The Netherlands   Internet: www.europe-on-the-move.nl

2. PUBLICATIONS

Please note: An extensive two-tier bibliography appends each of the contributions in this volume and includes a wide range of journals and monographs relating to physical activity and ageing. Resources listed at the end of each chapter are relevant to both specialists and non-specialists. Below is a list of selected journals and internet sites. Please refer to each chapter for monographs and additional specific resources.

2.1 Journals

- **Ageing Well**, journal of the National Ageing Research Institute, Australia.
- **Australasian Journal of Aging**, quarterly journal on ageing, Australia. <http://home.vicnet.net.au/~cotaa/aja.htm>
- **Journal of Aging and Health**, quarterly journal, University of Texas, USA <www.sagepub.co.uk/journals/details/j0100.html>
- **Journal of Aging and Physical Activity**, official quarterly journal of ISAPA
- **Journal of the American Geriatrics Society**, AGS Official monthly journal
- **Journal of the British Geriatrics Society**, Oxford University Press, U.K. <www.bgs.org.uk/publications.htm>
- **Journal of Women and Aging**, Haworth Press, NY, USA, abstracts available online <http://bubl.ac.uk/journals/soc/jwaa/>
- **Medicine & Science in Sports & Exercise** (MSSE), official Journal of the American College of Sports Medicine, monthly journal, Keyword: geriatrics.

2.2 Position Statements

Exercise and physical activity in older persons. American College of Sports Medicine Position Stand. *Medical Science in Sports and Exercise* (US), Jun 1998, 30(6) pp. 992-1008.
<http://www.com/MSSE/0195-91316-98p992.html>

The Heidelberg Guidelines for Promoting Physical Activity among Older Persons. World Health Organization. (1996).
These guidelines were prepared by a scientific committee and submitted to participants at the 4th International Congress on Physical Activity, Ageing and Sports (Heidelberg, Germany, August 1996).
<http://www.who.dk/zoro/inv/aging.htm>

3. INTERNET RESOURCES

3.1 Directories

Journals on Ageing
<http://crab.rutgers.edu/~deppen/journals.htm>
A comprehensive directory of geriatrics/gerontology with periodical literature available on ageing and health care has been compiled by Monica Deppen Wood of Rutgers University, Camden, NJ, USA. It also aims to assist researchers and academics from various disciplines in selecting appropriate journals as they seek to publish their work. All journals focus primarily on ageing and/or on health care of older individuals.

Health and Ageing
<www.genevaassociation.org/health-newsletter.htm>
An extensive list of books, journals, abstracts and international organisations compiled by The Geneva Association, a unique world organisation formed by some 80 Chief Executive Officers of the most important insurance companies in Western Europe, the United States and Japan.

Health Knowledge Network and Medical Library
<http://www.med.ucalgary.ca/>

This database lets you search indexes of the world's health sciences literature.

MedWEB
<www.medweb.emory.edu>
Biomedical Internet Resources, Emory University, Atlanta, Georgia, USA.
This searchable site provides biomedical information, services and technology to improve education, research and patient care. Recommended search by Keyword: Geriatrics.

Sport Quest
<http://www.SPORTQuest.com/>
An easy-to-use searchable directory of sport websites and full text covering topics such as sports medicine, physical fitness and coaching.

WHO Active Living Resources
<http://www.who.int/hpr/active/ref.html>
A bibliography of relevant publications and WHO documents.

SIRC Conference Calendar
<www.SPORTQuest.com/sirc/calen.html>
A current list of forthcoming international congresses, conferences, symposia, and seminars dealing with sport science and physical education. Updated weekly.

3.2   Additional Resources in Alphabetical Order
(many include information in multiple languages)

Action for healthy ageing and elderly care
<http://www.healthandage.com/>
The Novartis Gerontology Foundation supports education and innovation in geriatric medicine, general practice, supportive care and patient management to prevent dysfunction in later life.

American Heart Association (AHA)

A wealth of information on heart health, research, health promotion, prevention, treatment, and recovery, as well as a cross reference index to heart and stroke related matters.

The Centre for Activity and Ageing
<www.uwo.ca/actage/about.html>
This Centre at the University of Western Ontario, Canada combines research investigation of the interrelationship of physical activity and ageing, and the translation of research findings into strategies in order to maintain the ageing population in independent lifestyles, or to maintain or improve the functional levels of those living in a more dependent environment.

Centre on Aging
<http://www.coag.uvic.ca/>
This multidisciplinary research centre at the University of Victoria in Victoria, B.C., Canada, promotes and conducts basic and applied research throughout the lifespan, and produces a newsletter and public access to its resource library.

Cooper Institute for Aerobics Research
<http://www.cooperinst.org/>
The Cooper Institute in Dallas, Texas, USA, is one of the leaders in preventive medicine research and education dedicated to advancing the understanding of the relationship between living habits and health, and providing leadership in implementing these concepts to enhance the physical and emotional well-being of individuals.

Council on Aging
<http://coa.ottawa.com/>
A bilingual, non-profit voluntary organisation in Ottawa-Carleton, Canada, that deals with the concerns of senior citizens, particularly in health, education and social issues to voice issues and concerns to all levels of government and the general public.

Duke University Diet and Fitness Center
<www.dukecenter.org/dfc/>
The Duke Center for Living in Durham, North Carolina, USA, is composed of several programs for wellness and better living, including weight loss, health

and personal wellness, as well as rehabilitation for arthritis and cardiac and pulmonary disorders.

Fifty-Plus Net, Canadian Association of Retired Persons (CARP)
<www.fifty-plus.net>
A Canadian online community providing unique content, health, fitness and advocacy for the needs of the over-fifty population (incl. forums and chat rooms).

National Ageing Research Institute (NARI)
Affiliated with the University of Melbourne in Australia.

The National Insitute on Aging (NIA)
<www.nih.gov/nia/>
Federal Effort on Aging Research in USA with 25 institutes and centers to understand the nature of aging and to extend the healthy, active years of life.

National Coalition for Promoting Physical Activity
<http://www.a1.com/ncppa/>
A collaborative partnership to unite and inspire Americans to lead physically active and healthy lifestyles with several NCPPA related links to organisations, reports, alerts, and program options for effective action at the state and community levels.

Physical Activity and Health: A Report of the Surgeon General
<http://www.cdc.gov/nccdphp/sgr/sgr.htm>
This site includes the Report's executive summary, contents, fact sheets, related information and ordering information.

UKK Institute for Health Promotion of Health Enhancing Physical Activity (HEPA)
<www.europa.eu.int/comm/health/ph/programmes/health/network5.htm>
The general aim of this project is to further the promotion of health enhancing physical activity (HEPA) in Europe by strengthening the "Europe on the Move!" HEPA network and by promoting walking.

ICSSPE

CIEPSS

International Council of Sport Science and Physical Education (ICSSPE)

Join ICSSPE!

If your organisation wishes to:
➢ Benefit from the experience of others
➢ Contribute its own experience for the benefit of others
➢ Become part of the international network of physical education and sport science,

Join the International Council of Sport Science and Physical Education!
ICSSPE admits members in four categories:
A) Governmental organisations and non-governmental bodies that are the major organisations responsible for sport or sport science in their respective countries.
B) International organisations working to unify, co-ordinate, and promote activities in the field of physical education and sport: (a) international organisations concerned with sport science, physical education, sport and recreation; (b) international sport federations; (c) international organisations (cultural, artistic, scientific) with an interest in sport and physical education.
C) National non-governmental organisations concerned with sport science, physical education, sport and recreation.
D) Research institutes and schools of higher learning in physical education or sport science.

Currently more than 220 organisations and institutions form all parts of the world are affiliated with ICSSPE.

Please contact the Executive Office for more information:

ICSSPE/CIEPSS
Am Kleinen Wannsee 6
14109 Berlin
GERMANY

Tel. +49 30 805 00360
Fax +49 30 805 6386
E-mail: icsspe@icsspe.or
Internet: www.icsspe.org

Our first volume
of Perspectives

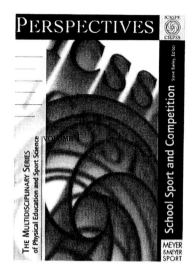

ICSSPE (International Council of Sport Science and Physical Education)

Perspectives: The Multidisciplinary Series of Physical Education and Sport Science
Volume 1

School Sport and Competition

State of the art themes are addressed by sport science specialists from numerous different discipline areas. The first volume of this one of a kind multidisciplinary monograph series focuses on competition in school sports. Sport scientists present perspectives from the fields of sport psychology, pedagogy, adapted physical activity, management, facility planning and physiology. Ms. Anita DeFrantz, IOC Vice-President, opens the publication with a personal commentary. A detailed information section, including contact addresses and internet resources concludes the publication.

144 pages, 14 photos and figures
paperback, 14.8 x 21 cm
ISBN: 1-84126-019-3
£ 14.95 UK/$ 19.95 US/$ 29.95 Cdn

MEYER & MEYER Verlag | Von-Coels-Straße 390 | D-52080 Aachen | Fax + + 49 (0)2 41/9 58 10-10

11/00

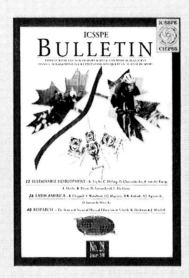